Pig Disease Identification and Diagnosis Guide

NEWTON R G

Pig Disease Identification and Diagnosis Guide

Steven McOrist BVSc PhD

Consultant Pig Veterinarian

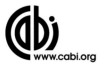

www.cabi.org

CABI is a trading name of CAB International

CABI
Nosworthy Way
Wallingford
Oxfordshire OX10 8DE
UK

CABI
38 Chauncy Street
Suite 1002
Boston, MA 02111
USA

Tel: +44 (0)1491 832111
Fax: +44 (0)1491 833508
E-mail: info@cabi.org
Website: www.cabi.org

Tel: +1 800 552 3083 (toll free)
Tel: +1 (0)617 395 4051
E-mail: cabi-nao@cabi.org

A catalogue record for this book is available from the British Library, London, UK.

Library of Congress Cataloging-in-Publication Data

McOrist, Steven, author.
  Pig disease identification and diagnosis guide / Steven McOrist.
    p. ; cm.
  Includes index.
  ISBN 978-1-78064-212-3 (hbk. : alk. paper) -- ISBN 978-1-78064-462-2
(pbk. : alk. paper)
  I. C.A.B. International, issuing body. II. Title.
  [DNLM: 1. Swine Diseases--diagnosis--Case Reports. 2. Diagnosis, Differential--Case Reports. SF 971]

  SF971
  636.4'0896--dc23

                                        2014002484

ISBN-13: 978 1 78064 212 3 (hbk)
ISBN-13: 978 1 78064 462 2 (pbk)

Commissioning editor: Julia Killick
Editorial assistant: Alexandra Lainsbury
Production editor: Shankari Wilford

Typeset by SPi, Pondicherry, India
Printed and bound by Gutenberg Press Limited, Tarxien, Malta

Contents

Introduction

The aim of this book is to enhance problem recognition skills on pig farms. The book contains a series of cases involving either management faults or a clinical sign on the farm, such as reproductive problems, diarrhoea, coughing or lameness. This format of personal engagement with a case study and questions, followed by some comments and further scientific thoughts, is now considered the best approach for readers to learn the intended problem-solving skills.

There are two main problems with this type of approach. First, providing a set of cases does not easily imply priority or prevalence. Diseases such as swine fever or pneumonia can be much more likely or more severe in some regions than others. So the reader has to also consider local prevalence – this information is gained from industry leaders and the diagnostic steps during an investigation. The second problem with this approach is the limitations of the static picture format for case illustration, as compared with viewing a case study in reality or on a video. Static pictures will never be particularly dramatic to illustrate pigs that are coughing, are lame or are showing nervous signs.

Pig farms are classified in this book as breeder farms or production farms. A typical pig farm system consists of three separate areas: (i) one for breeding practices (mating, gestation or pregnancy, farrowing and lactation); (ii) one for the weaning or nursery period from 3 to 10 weeks old; and (iii) a fattening or finishing area, where pigs grow from 10 weeks old to marketing weight.

The details of the cases that ended up in this book were formulated over the past 35 years of my life in Pig Land, during discussions with a wide range of people. Some of these great people, who also hopefully enjoyed the discussions about pig cases, include Roberta Alvarez, Brad Bosworth, Enrique Corona, Mark Hammer, Tim Klein, Gerardo Iglesias, Paul Pattison, Jomar Percil, Les Sims, Daniel Spiru and Mark White.

Some of the pictures in this book were kindly contributed by the following people: John Carr, Tony Fahy, Brook Fang, K. Khampee, Liz Lloyd and Daniel Spiru.

Steven McOrist
Consultant Pig Veterinarian
BVSc (Melbourne)
PhD (Edinburgh)
Diplomate, European College of Veterinary Pathology
Diplomate, European College of Pig Health and Management

Abbreviations

AI	artificial insemination
APP	*Actinobacillus pleuropneumoniae*
ASF	African swine fever
CH_4	methane
CO	carbon monoxide
CSF	classical swine fever
DDGS	dried distiller's grains with solubles
ESF	electronic sow feeding
ETEC	enterotoxigenic *Escherichia coli*
FMD	foot-and-mouth disease
HEV	haemagglutinating encephalitis virus
HPS	*Haemophilus parasuis*
H_2S	hydrogen sulfide
IU	international units
JE	Japanese encephalitis
NBA	number of piglets born alive
NH_3	ammonia
OGU	oesophageal gastric ulceration
OIE	World Organisation for Animal Health
PCV-2	porcine circovirus 2
PDNS	porcine dermatopathy and nephropathy syndrome
PED	porcine epidemic diarrhoea
PHE	proliferative haemorrhagic enteropathy
PMWS	post-weaning multi-systemic wasting syndrome
PPV	porcine parvovirus
PRDC	porcine respiratory disease complex
PRRS	porcine reproductive and respiratory syndrome
SD	swine dysentery
SOP	standard operating procedure
SVD	swine vesicular disease
TGE	transmissible gastroenteritis

PART 1
Management Problems on Pig Farms

1.1   Case Study

The farmer operated a nursery and finisher pig farm system, with groups of finisher pigs kept in a variety of indoor and outdoor pens. Some groups of finisher pigs were raised in open-plan sheds with canvas roofs and the floors consisting of soil and bedding materials (Fig. 1.1i). The farmer used a variety of sources of bedding materials, such as straw, cereal husks and waste horticulture materials. Pig were raised in these sheds from 25 to 100 kg bodyweight, and then sent for slaughter. The farmer obtained the weaner pigs at 25 kg bodyweight, from a modern breeder farm. The finisher pigs were generally alert and eating well, but some groups were thought to be uneven in growth. The pigs did not have any cough or diarrhoea problems. The farmer was called by the operator of the local slaughterhouse, following the delivery of a truck-load of 100–110 kg pigs. During the processing of the pigs, the slaughterhouse workers were shocked to see some enormous worms inside the small intestines (Fig. 1.1ii). They also noticed most of the livers of these pigs had multi-focal fibrotic lesions, which looked like someone had dropped some spots of milk on to the livers.

Key Features

- Pig production in settings with soil-and-bedding floors.
- Large worms in the intestines and milk spots on the liver.

1.1a. What is this problem?

1.1b. What control measures may assist the herd?

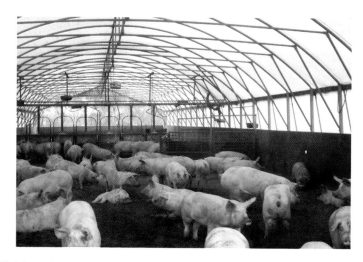

Fig. 1.1i. Finisher pigs in open-plan sheds with soil-and-bedding floors.

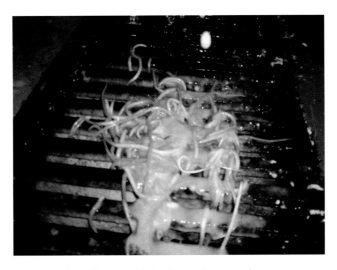

Fig. 1.1ii.   Large worms from the small intestines at processing.

1.1   Comments

1.1a. This is intestinal parasitism due to the large pig nematode worm *Ascaris suum*. Its life cycle inside the pig includes larval worm movement through the liver and lungs, then worm maturity in the pig intestines. The larval movements of *A. suum* in the liver is the cause of the 'milk spot' liver lesions. There is a period of 4–5 weeks between the pig eating a worm egg that is contained in the residual faecal material in the soil and bedding material on the ground, until the worm becomes an adult in the pig intestines. This period is known as the pre-patent period. The overall incidence of these worms in pigs declined greatly with construction and population of modern indoor farms in the 1970s, with raised, slatted-concrete floors, which breaks the oral–faecal infection cycle. However, the incidence of pig worms is now increasing again and is significantly higher in outdoor farm systems. Infection of farm sites only requires a small number of infected pigs to enter the site, during an initial stocking with pigs from variable sources. The thick-coated *A. suum* eggs are then highly stable and infectious in the environment of soil-and-bedding farm floor systems for several years. It is also likely that farm equipment and wild birds may also act to spread the eggs around a farm site. The presence of the larval worm lesions in the liver (milk spot liver) and lungs may result in a downgrading of the price of the pigs for the farmer.

1.1b. Farms that have been infected for some time should employ ongoing medication programmes. Treatment usually involves delivery of an anthelminthic medication via the feed or water supply. Routine anthelminthic benzimidazoles (such as flubendazole) or ivermectins are adequate – resistance of the worms to drugs has not been a major issue. The timing of medication for *A suum* is generally aimed to prevent mature intestinal infection. This is achieved by medicating finisher pigs at intervals of 4 weeks apart.

The cleaning of farm sites for ascarid eggs is generally not practical. In outdoor pig systems, where pigs are kept on pastures, careful attention must be paid to stock management, with field rotations, low stocking densities and regular anthelminthic treatments.

1.2 Case Study

The farmer operated a medium-sized grower and finisher pig farm, which was constructed in an isolated and open-landscape situation. The farmer and some casual staff had installed all the electrical and mechanical ventilation systems in the farm buildings. The pigs were generally healthy and received a complete vaccination programme. The region had cold winters and warm summers, with many thunderstorms in the spring. During a large storm at night-time, the farm was hit by lightning strikes. The following day the farmer opened the doors of the unit to find a very large number of the finisher pigs were dead. Close inspection indicated that the room was very hot, and all the dead pigs were dirty and smelly (Fig. 1.2i). Many of the dead pigs were rotten and full of gas. The death rate was estimated at 90–95%, with the only surviving pigs being the smallest ones in the group. Large burns were evident on the main electrical systems controlling the mechanical ventilation systems and they did not function properly (Fig. 1.2ii).

Key Features

- Faults with the mechanical equipment used to control the indoor environment.
- Multiple deaths of larger pigs indoors.

1.2a. What is this problem?
1.2b. What are the important management systems required to prevent this problem?

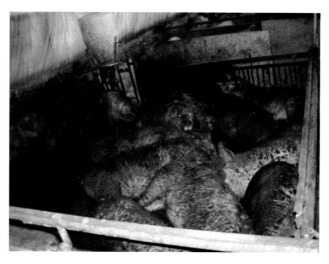

Fig. 1.2i. Groups of dirty and smelly dead finisher pigs.

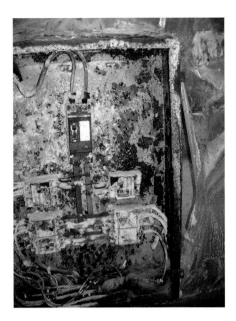

Fig. 1.2ii. Damaged farm-building electrical system.

1.2 Comments

1.2a. This death of larger pigs inside an enclosed room is due to excess heat, in a process known as hyperthermia. The housing of pigs inside enclosed rooms assists biosecurity and allows pigs to be raised throughout the year, even in regions with cold winters. However, any fault and cause of electrical or machine-related stoppage (such as a lightning strike) to the ventilation systems will result in the mechanical heating or cooling systems to cease functioning. This will lead to the consequent loss of cooling ventilation in the affected building. Heat rapidly builds up inside the building as a result of the presence of many larger pigs inside the room and will quickly result in this pig hyperthermia situation and many deaths of pigs in the enclosed buildings.

1.2b. The pig does not have many innate systems to control its body temperature, as they do not sweat (except from the snout). Therefore in hot conditions, pigs must be supplied with cooling ventilation or water cooling systems. Water cooling systems, such as drip lines, mist-spray devices or shallow pools in pens, allow the pig to lose heat via the cooling effect of water evaporation on the skin. However, in some tropical climates with high humidity, the water will not evaporate and the pigs will not be cooled. The growth performance of pigs in open buildings in tropical climates is therefore unlikely to match those in temperate climates.

In pigs housed in enclosed buildings, any fault or cause of electrical or machine-related stoppage (such as lightning strike) to the mechanical ventilation systems will result in the hyperthermia situation inside enclosed buildings. Therefore great attention must be given to correct installation of lightning rod and electrical earthing systems, and the operation of electrical- and mechanical-fault warning alarm systems on farms. These alarm systems should be tested each week on the farm. Other management factors to keeping pigs comfortable in housed accommodation include: (i) adequate insulation linings; (ii) high volumes of water flow in drinkers; and (iii) low stocking rates.

1.3 Case Study

The farmer operated an established nursery and finisher farm, with grower pigs housed in a variety of older-style buildings. The pigs had a range of general problems such as diarrhoea, coughing and lameness, but none of these problems was considered particularly serious. Some of the pens in the older buildings had older, poorly maintained floors. On some occasions, the farmer received and housed larger numbers of pigs to maintain throughput of finisher pig numbers. In some pens of grower pigs, the farmer noticed blood on the faces of many pigs, and a few pigs in these pens had bloody protrusions from their backside. Close inspection indicated that these affected younger grower pigs had a portion of their intestines protruding in a bloody mass oozing out from the anus, in a condition known as a rectal prolapse (Fig. 1.3i). Examination of the older pigs in the finisher areas on the farm also revealed that occasional pigs had a large swollen abdomen appearance, looking like a 'pot-belly'. These pot-belly pigs were small and hairy with a prominent ridged spine (Fig. 1.3ii).

Key Features

- Prolapse of rectum from anus of grower pigs.
- Pot-belly pigs noted in finisher areas.

1.3a. What is this problem?
1.3b. What control measures may assist the herd?

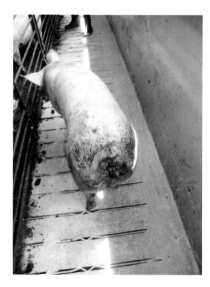

Fig. 1.3i. Grower pig with rectal prolapse.

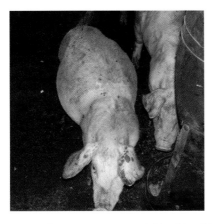

Fig. 1.3ii. Finisher pig with pot-belly appearance and thin ridged back.

1.3　Comments

1.3a. The problem in the groups of younger grower pigs is prolapse of the rectum, where the pig has pushed the terminal part of its own intestine outside of the body, via the anus. It is not an infectious problem, but it is a common event in pigs in farms around the world. There are many suggested risk factors for an increased incidence of rectal prolapse on farms, but cases often appear sporadically and it is difficult to place an exact cause and effect. The suggested risk factors include: (i) overcrowding of pigs in pens and trucks; (ii) excess feed intake and excess dietary lysine; (iii) a short tail length; (iv) diarrhoea; (v) coughing; (vi) straining to defecate; (vii) older sloping floors; and (viii) lameness problems.

If a pig suffers a rectal prolapse and the rectum is not repaired, then the protruding portion of intestine may be damaged or partially eaten by other pigs and the injury around the anus will heal by fibrous scar tissue. This will lead to a restriction of the rectal and anus openings, known as a rectal stricture. These pigs with rectal stricture will not defecate properly and will have a swollen abdomen full of poorly digested food and constipation – these are the pot-belly pigs in the older groups of finisher pigs. These pigs are generally culled from the herd.

1.3b. The management of a recently prolapsed rectum in an individual pig entails examination of the prolapse to determine if it is suitable to be replaced back into the pig. The prolapse is often swollen and bloody, but should not be replaced if it is necrotic or torn. The pig should be sedated and the hindquarters raised upwards. The prolapse should be washed and cleaned and gently re-positioned with the hands. The prolapse is then held in place with a one-finger anal opening and a purse-string circular suture placed around the anal ring. This suture should be removed after 5 days. Failure to provide surgery will lead to the cannibalism and poor healing of the prolapse, with the rectal stricture problem occurring and likely culling of the pig.

It can be difficult to address all the suggested risk factors for rectal prolapse on a pig farm. Feed supply to pigs should be steady and constant, with no surges or interruptions. When tail docking or trimming is performed, it should consist of surgical removal of only a portion of the distal tail in neonatal piglets, to no fewer than three vertebrae adjacent to the trunk. The piglet is therefore left with a reasonable length of tail muscles to assist defecation. Floors should be even and properly maintained.

1.4   Case Study

The farmer operated an established medium-sized grower and finisher pig unit, in which he had constructed various open-sided and enclosed buildings. The pen floors were concrete and the pen walls were constructed with local supplies of metal rods and sheets (Fig. 1.4i). The farmer had also installed all the farm electrical systems in open, exposed areas of the buildings (Fig. 1.4ii). The farm pigs were generally healthy and the pens were vigorously cleaned and disinfected between batches. The farm suffered periods of windy and rainy weather. The farmer entered the farm one day to find several of the grower pigs lying dead, in a group of metal-sided pens in one area of a building. Close inspection indicated that some of these dead pigs had dark linear burn marks on their skin. Many of the other pigs in these pens appeared to be severely lame, with fractures to the bones of their legs and some were paralysed in the back legs and sitting down. At autopsy of the dead pigs, the farmer and veterinarian noticed that the body organs appeared congested, with large haemorrhages on the heart and skeletal muscles.

Key Features

- Faults with the electrical circuits in the farm.
- Multiple deaths and bone fractures of pigs in one location.

1.4a. What is this problem?
1.4b. What are the important management systems required to prevent this problem?

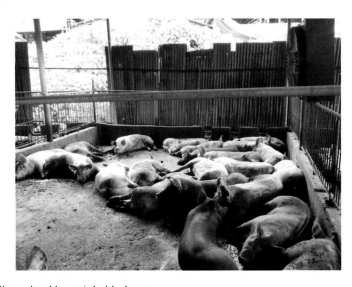

Fig. 1.4i. Pigs raised in metal-sided pens.

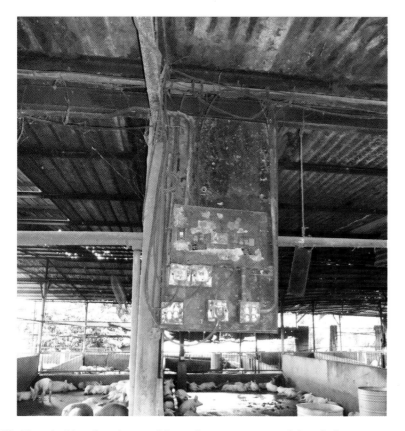

Fig. 1.4ii. Electrical box for wires and fuses in an open area of the pig farm.

1.4   Comments

1.4a. This is a case study of deaths and bone fractures due to electrocution of pigs, which have come into contact with live wires and/or metal pens. This type of electrocution of pigs or humans is a relatively common event on pig farms, often due to faulty or home-made electrical wiring and plugs. Many plugs and electrical fittings can deteriorate over time, particularly in situations where they may be repeatedly exposed to powerful washing and cleaning practices for pig-farm hygiene purposes. Any lack of attention to these possible problems with electrical circuits can lead to consequent overloading and fusing of any electrical circuits, with the wires or contact metal-pen areas becoming live with electrical current. This will cause the electrocution of any group of pigs that come into contact with the electrical fault area, such as metal-sided pens with wet floors.

If it is suspected that any pig might have been subject to electrocution it is obviously vital that the local electrical power is turned off, prior to any handling of the affected electrified pigs by farm workers.

1.4b. Great attention must be given to correct installation and maintenance of the electrical plugs, wires and fittings on farms. Any indoor electrical fittings that are washed regularly must be maintained and replaced, whenever they appear damaged.

1.5 Case Study

The farmer operated an established farm system with breeder, nursery and finisher units, with various older-style buildings. The breeder pigs and young piglets all received a complete vaccination programme. However, the farmer did not complete a tail-docking or teeth-clipping programme. The breeding farm had a variety of modern pig breeds. These pig breeds had a rapid growth rate and some grower and finisher pig pens had became busy and overcrowded, particularly in some of the older buildings. The farmer noticed that among groups of these rapidly growing and vigorous grower pigs, there was limited feeder and movement space and the air flow seemed poor. Several of the pigs had noticeable tail wounds. Close inspection indicated the presence of bloody bite wounds and ulcers on the tails of several pigs in each pen (Fig. 1.5i). In some pigs, there was also bite and blood-filled wounds on the ears or vulva (Fig. 1.5ii). The tail wounds were noticed in many grower pigs in some pens, with lesions in various stages of being developed and chewed, with some deep ulcers around the base of the tail in more severe cases. In some older finisher pigs, the tail wounds had progressed to pus-filled abscess areas. Careful inspection of these groups of grower pigs located one or more aggressor pigs with blood on their faces and mouths, and normal long tails. Examination of the finisher pigs at the slaughterhouse confirmed the presence of many pigs with tail wounds and abscesses in the tail and spine areas.

Key Features

- Rapidly growing pigs in accommodation with limited space.
- Bite and attack wounds, particularly on the un-docked tails.

1.5a. What is this problem?
1.5b. What control measures may assist the herd?

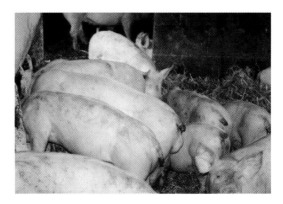

Fig. 1.5i. Group of grower pigs with biting lesions on the tail.

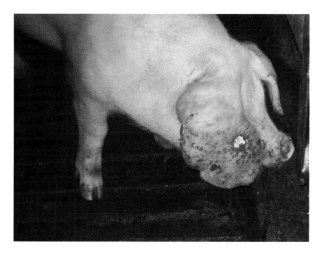

Fig. 1.5ii. Pig with biting and blood-filled lesions on the ears.

1.5 Comments

1.5a. This is tail-biting activity among groups of grower and finisher pigs. It is a common problem in pig farms around the world. The tip of the entire (un-docked) tail normally has a poor nerve supply and can be bitten by the aggressor pigs without much response by its owner. This behavioural problem can then become persistent and the aggressor pigs will continue to attack other pigs.

There are various suggested factors that predispose to this destructive behavioural habit commencing and persisting in a group of pigs. The main factors appear to be a combination of crowding among grower pigs and the existence of aggression among modern lines of pig breeds. Some lines of pigs have strong aggressive and biting tendencies towards other group members and also farm staff. This can be more obvious and manifest in herd problems in buildings and pens with high stocking density and poor air flow. It is also more likely in situations with high and constant lighting levels – the tail is more visible in front of the aggressor pig. It is also likely that many of these pigs enjoy the taste of meat and blood, particularly since meat and bonemeal ingredients have been removed from the grower and finisher pig diets in many countries.

1.5b. The aggressor pigs need to be identified and removed and the light levels should be lowered in the affected pens. If the injuries are not severe, they can be treated with antibiotic sprays and injections and the application of bitter-tasting spray to the tails.

Many scientific studies have concluded that tail docking reduces the incidence of tail biting in pigs. The tip of the undocked tail normally has a poor enervation and can be bitten by other pigs without much response. The fact that the tail-docked pig is less likely to have a bitten tail is therefore explained by the presence of sensitive nerve endings in the docked tail-end. Any tail-docked pig that is 'nibbled' is likely to have a quickened response and will naturally attempt to repel the aggressor pig. Tail docking or trimming usually consists of surgical removal of a portion of the distal tail in neonatal piglets, to no fewer than three vertebrae adjacent to the trunk. Tail docking should be done at 1–5 days of age, but not before 6 hours of age. The use of sharp and specialized instruments with good antiseptic hygiene and wound dressing are vital.

1.6 Case Study

The farmer operated an established medium-sized grower and finisher pig farm, with various open-sided and enclosed buildings. The pens were constructed with local supplies of materials. The farmer had also constructed a variety of feeder supply systems for the pens. In some pens, solid feed was placed directly into troughs by farm workers, and in other pens, feed-storage hopper bins were placed above the troughs. The farmer was concerned about feed costs and ordered solid feed from a local feed mill in sporadic batches. The pigs were generally healthy and received a complete vaccination programme. The farmer had few staff and maintenance of the farm buildings was not adequate. The farmer noticed that the time required for groups of pigs to reach slaughter weight was getting longer. Close inspection of the farm feed orders, the weights of the pigs and of the number of days for the pigs to grow from weaning date to slaughter weight indicated that the feed intake of the pigs was below target levels. Inspection of the farm pens indicated many feeders had blockages and spillages (Fig. 1.6i). Many pigs in these pens appeared small for their age and gathered around feeders (Fig. 1.6ii). The farmer had also reported some pigs dying suddenly, with bloated abdomens, due to intestinal twists and torsions.

Key Features

- Slow growth rates in production pigs.
- Faults with the feeders on the farm.

1.6a. What is this problem?
1.6b. What are the important management systems required to prevent this problem?

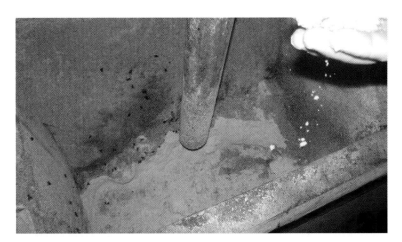

Fig. 1.6i. Pig feeder with a blockage.

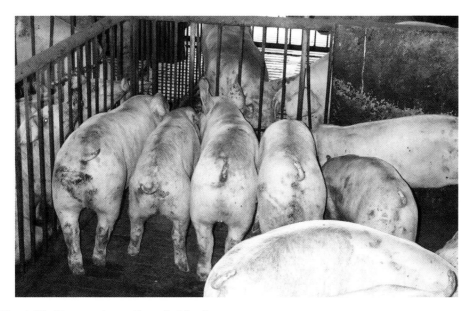

Fig. 1.6ii. Hungry pigs gathered at feeders.

1.6 Comments

1.6a. This is a problem of insufficient feed intake by groups of production pigs, leading to slow growth rates. Confirmation of this problem requires close inspection of a representative batch of pigs, for their feed intake and growth rate, which is checked via weighing some pigs. An average pig will eat 210–220 kg feed from 4 weeks old to 21 weeks old. The amount of feed that is ordered and stored also needs to be assessed. Problems with the ordering and storage of feed and problems with the actual feeding arrangements for the pens are common on pig farms around the world. The actual feed supply in the troughs in the pens of pigs needs to be monitored daily by staff and/or electrical recording. Some common problems are: (i) over-ordering of feed, leading to feed stores with excess stale feed; (ii) poor hygiene and poor maintenance of stores and feed mixers, troughs and hopper bins, leading to feed supply blockages; and (iii) quick changes and mixing of feed supply between younger and older pigs.

When feed supply has been reduced but is then reintroduced to a group of pigs, sudden deaths due to intestinal torsion are commonly seen, probably due to rapid over-eating by the active pigs.

1.6b. The economics of pig farming involve the fact that feed costs are the highest proportion of the costs of raising a production pig. However, farmers should enable all pigs to eat adequately throughout their life. Pig farms should: (i) review feed-ordering protocols; (ii) check that a clean feed supply is constantly available to all pigs; and (iii) ensure that all stores, mixers and delivery equipment are well maintained. The feeder equipment should be cleaned between each large batch of pigs, or twice a year. Changes in the diets of pigs should be made gradually, particularly for younger pigs.

The water supply points (nipples or bowls) for pens should be placed close to the feeder supply points. Pigs tend to stop eating and take a drink then return to eating. If the water points are poorly placed, then they will not return to eat as readily.

1.7   Case Study

The farmer operated an established nursery and finisher pig farm system, with older-style buildings. The farmer also did a lot of construction work and had a lot of extraneous building waste equipment and materials around the farm site (Fig. 1.7i). The groups of grower and finisher pigs were raised in large groups in open-plan pens with floors consisting of soil and bedding materials. The pigs were generally healthy and received a complete vaccination programme. The farmer used a variety of sources of bedding materials, such as straw, cereal husks, waste horticulture materials and waste construction materials. The farmer noticed that some of the finisher pigs were sick (Fig. 1.7ii). Close inspection indicated that occasional pigs were dull, depressed and not eating well. Some of these pigs appeared to have a yellow colour to their skin and had become recumbent. At autopsy of these few sick pigs, the farmer and veterinarian noticed that the skin and fat tissue was yellow (jaundice), the liver appeared enlarged and mottled, and there was a lot of fluid in the body cavities.

Key Features

- Pigs raised on variety of bedding materials.
- Sick pigs with liver changes.

1.7a. What is this problem?

1.7b. What are the important management systems required to prevent this problem?

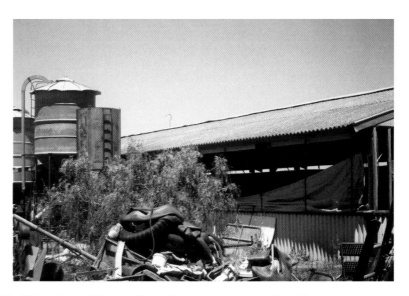

Fig. 1.7i. Older-style buildings with waste materials around the site.

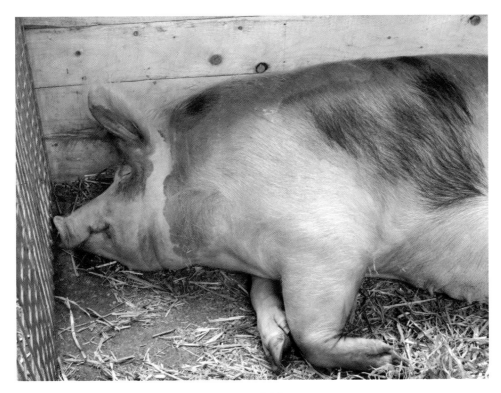

Fig. 1.7ii. Sick pig in a pen with bedding-material floors.

1.7 Comments

1.7a. This is illness and liver damage in pigs due to the intake of poisonous materials. The poison in this case study is likely to be phenol derived from coal tar. Coal tar is a component of waste from fence, roof, flooring and road materials and may be present on floors of pig pens and in bedding materials. Poisoning is not a common problem on most pig farms, but this phenol poison is probably the most common one involved in incidents in pigs housed indoors. Other poisonous chemicals kept on pig farms commonly include rodent poisons, crop and livestock chemicals, such as organophosphates, used for pest and insect control.

Studies of poisoning of pigs raised on pastures indicate that they will become sick if they have access to and eat poisonous weeds such as bracken fern (*Pteridium aquilinum*) or hemlock (*Conium maculatum*).

1.7b. It is vital to label all toxic chemicals properly and exclude all of them from around any feed preparation or mixing operation. It is also vital that any pigs raised outdoors do not have access to bracken fern or other poisonous plants.

1.8   Case Study

The farmer operated a medium-sized breeder, nursery and finisher pig farm system on a single site. The farmer maintained a good vaccination and medication programme for the pigs. The farmer also operated a feed-mixing and preparation facility on the same site, supplying all the different stages of feeds for the pigs. The farmer used local suppliers of feed ingredients, such as whole-maize (corn) cereals, soybeans and bio-fuel distillation by-products. Supplies of these items were stored at the farm and incorporated in various mixtures for each batch of feed. The farmer noticed that around 10–15% of young grower pigs on a new batch of feed, did not eat it properly (Fig. 1.8i). Close inspection indicated that these pigs went to the feeders, but did not consume the new feed offered. Some of the pigs in the group that were eating this new feed were salivating excessively and some had vomited the feed. Many of the pigs in this group looked in poor condition and some were found to have stomach ulcers. There was no noticeable coughing or diarrhoea. The farmer inspected the feed and maize cereals used to prepare the feed and noticed that much of the feed was damp and formed into crusty cakes, with some areas of dark mould evident on the feed and on the maize ingredients (Fig. 1.8ii). The farmer then purchased some fresh feed supplies without any moulds and the pigs ate this normally.

Key Features

- Mouldy feed supplies.
- Feed refusal in production pigs.

1.8a. What is this problem?
1.8b. What are the important management systems required to prevent this problem?

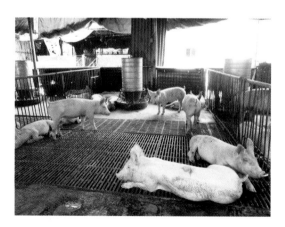

Fig. 1.8i. Pigs in poor condition and not eating.

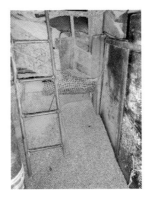

Fig. 1.8ii. Farm storage of maize with mould.

1.8   Comments

1.8a. This is a problem with feed refusal by groups of production pigs on mouldy feed. Moulds or fungi can readily grow on feed ingredients in warm and damp conditions. Mycotoxins comprise a chemically diverse group of secondary metabolites of moulds. Some of these moulds produce specific mycotoxins that are harmful to pigs. One of the more common forms of mycotoxin problem is illustrated in this case study. The Fusarium mould grows on maize and produces a mycotoxin called trichothecene or T2. The usual effect of this mycotoxin is for the sensitive pigs to refuse to eat the contaminated feed, with occasional vomiting. Confirmation of this problem requires close inspection of a representative batch of pigs, for their feed intake and growth rate check via weighing some pigs. During the last decade, the occurrence of mycotoxins in feed materials has probably increased, most probably as a result of changes in agricultural practice (i.e. pre-harvest contamination) and the use of new feed materials, particularly the increasing use of distillation residues known as dried distiller's grains with solubles (DDGS), from biofuel production from maize. The DDGS components can accumulate mycotoxins during their processing (postharvest contamination), prior to being packaged and added to animal feed.

1.8b. The feed problem can be eliminated by preparing and offering feed that is free of mycotoxins. Pigs are considered among the most sensitive animal species to the adverse effects of mycotoxins and hence recommendations for maximum levels of mycotoxins in feed ingredients and commercial animal feeds are widely known and checked to prevent intoxications in animals.

However, it can be difficult to eliminate all mycotoxins from feed, and moulds may develop during feed storage, prior to being fed to the pigs. Many pig farms therefore also use products added to the feed, known as mycotoxin inhibitors. These products are of two main types. The adsorbent type of mycotoxin inhibitor in feed consists of earthen chelate materials that act to bind and absorb the mould toxins, making them neutral to the pig. The second type of inhibitor is the microbial digester enzyme type that acts to break down the toxin in the pig's intestines. The adsorbent type of mycotoxin inhibitor tends to act more quickly and efficiently.

Most of the known mycotoxins have a short biological half-life and do not accumulate in animal tissues. They are therefore not a hazard for consumers of pig meats.

1.9 Case Study

The farmer operated a medium-sized breeder farm system with breeder females and boars on a single site. The farmer maintained a good vaccination and medication programme for the pigs. The farmer also operated a feed-mixing and preparation facility on the same site, supplying all the different stages of feeds for the pigs. The farmer used local suppliers of feed ingredients, such as whole-maize (corn) cereals, soybeans and biofuel distillation by-products. Supplies of these items were stored at the farm and incorporated in various mixtures for each batch of feed. The farmer raised the breeder pigs in large open pens with straw bedding. The farmer noticed that the results for the farrowing rates and the litter size and numbers born alive were becoming more variable, over a period of weeks. The farm workers also reported the occurrence of some abortions of whole dead litters in late pregnancy. Close inspection of breeding farm data confirmed a range of problems with fertility in the breeding herd, including: (i) failures to come into oestrous; (ii) lower conception rates (Fig. 1.9i); (iii) reduced number of piglets per litter; (iv) abortions; and (v) increased stillbirths. Examination of the farm boars showed some enlargement and reddening of their nipples and testicles. Examination of female suckling piglets also showed some enlargement and reddening of their vulvas. The farmer inspected the pen bedding and the pig feed and maize cereals and noticed that much of the straw and feed was damp and mouldy with some areas of dark mould evident on the straw bedding and pig feed and on the maize ingredients (Fig. 1.9ii).

Key Features

- Mouldy feed and straw-bedding supplies.
- Range of fertility problems.

1.9a. What is this problem?

1.9b. What are the important management systems required to prevent this problem?

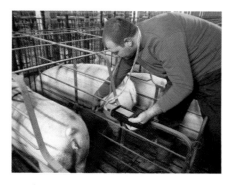

Fig. 1.9i. Pregnancy checks showing lack of conception.

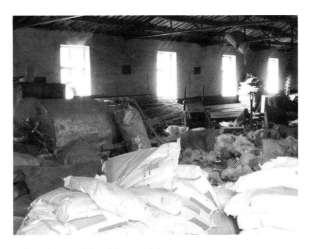

Fig. 1.9ii. Storage of maize and feed in mouldy area.

1.9 Comments

1.9a. This is a problem with fertility in groups of breeder pigs on mouldy feed and bedding. Moulds or fungi can readily grow on feed ingredients in warm and damp conditions. Some of these moulds produce specific mycotoxins that are harmful to pigs. Mycotoxins comprise a chemically diverse group of secondary metabolites of moulds. One of the more common forms of mycotoxin problem is illustrated in this case study. The Fusarium mould grows on maize and produces a mycotoxin called zearalenone or F-2. The usual effect of this mycotoxin is a hormonal or oestrogenic effect, resulting in disruption to oestrous cycles, pregnancy and genital organs. Confirmation of this problem requires close inspection of a representative batch of pigs, for their fertility. During the last decade, the occurrence of mycotoxins in feed materials has probably increased, most probably due to changes in agricultural practice (i.e. pre-harvest contamination) and also to the use of new feed materials, particularly the increasing use of distillation residues known as DDGS, from biofuel production from maize. The DDGS components can accumulate mycotoxins during their processing (postharvest contamination), prior to being packaged and added to animal feed.

1.9b. The problem can be eliminated by preparing and offering feed that is free of mycotoxins. Pigs are considered among the most sensitive animal species to the adverse effects of mycotoxins and hence recommendations for maximum levels of mycotoxins in feed ingredients and commercial animal feeds are widely known and checked to prevent intoxication in animals.

It can be difficult to eliminate all mycotoxins from feed and moulds may develop in feed storage prior to being fed to the pigs. Many pig farms therefore also use products known as mycotoxin inhibitors that are added to the feed. These are of two main types. The adsorbent type of mycotoxin inhibitor in feed consists of earthen chelate materials that act to bind and absorb the mould toxins, making them neutral to the pig. The second type of inhibitor is the microbial digester enzyme that acts to break down the toxin in the pig's intestines. The adsorbent type of mycotoxin inhibitor tends to act more quickly and efficiently.

1.10   Case Study

The farmer operated an established breeder farm, with various lines of breeder sows, with several boars for natural matings. The pigs received a complete vaccination programme. The farm buildings for the gilts and sows in the gestation and natural mating areas consisted of various old buildings and some outside pens next to these buildings. The floors in the pens and individual pig stalls were a mixture of solid concrete and some wooden structures. Some of the walkways and floors of breeder pens had poor drainage areas and had become rough and dirty over the years of use (Fig. 1.10i). The farmer had few staff and hygiene levels were low. The farm staff used a few old buckets and gloves to assist female pigs giving birth. In previous years, the farmer had noted that the annual rate of culling and mortality among the sow numbers was around 5%. However, in the current year, the overall annual mortality rate in the sows had risen to above 10%. Close inspection indicated that many sows had various types of noticeable vaginal discharges (Fig. 1.10ii). In some sows, these discharges occurred soon after farrowing. In other sows, the discharges occurred soon after weaning, that is soon after the natural matings with boars. The discharges generally consisted of noticeable amounts of messy and smelly grey and bloody slimy material, pouring from the vagina on to the floor of the pens.

Key Features

- Breeder pigs housed in dirty pens.
- Messy discharge from vulva of sows.

1.10a. What is this problem?
1.10b. What are the important management systems required to prevent this problem?

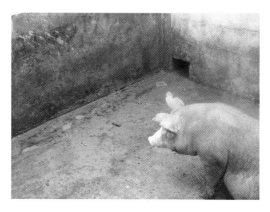

Fig. 1.10i. Breeder pigs in old and dirty pens.

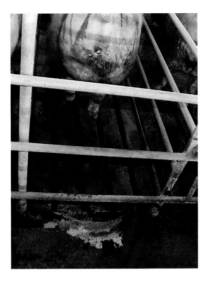

Fig. 1.10ii. Vaginal discharges from a sow.

1.10 Comments

1.10a. This problem is vaginal discharges, which are usually due to a bacterial infection in the lower part of the uterus. The infection occurs when environmental bacteria enter the vagina from the outside (e.g. faecal material in pens) and rise up into the uterus and start an infection, which produces some bloody pus and discharge materials. The bacteria that cause these infections are usually a range of environmental bacteria such as *Escherichia coli* or *Streptococcus* spp., with no specific strains involved. The occurrence of vaginal discharges is a common problem on many pig farms around the world. However, the problems are usually much more prominent in pigs raised on older established breeder farms with an overall level of poor hygiene. The housing of sows in stalls with solid wooden areas and solid boards at the rear of the sow makes cleaning difficult and retains faeces near the vagina of sows. To maintain proper hygiene on pig farms requires adequate staff and time.

The manual assistance of sows by staff by insertion of their arm into the birth canal, without the use of hygienic and clean gloves will lead to infections and discharges after farrowing. The service of sows by boars in mating pens that are not hygienic can result in infections after mating with dirty boars.

1.10b. Affected sows can be treated with antibiotics, but these sows can often suffer a recurrence and culling may be required. The farm hygiene needs to be improved, with better cleaning of all surfaces around sows and of the sows and boars themselves. In particular, faeces should not be allowed to accumulate at the rear of sows in stalls or pens. Also, assistance of sows at farrowing and mating needs to be performed in a hygienic manner with use of clean equipment, gloves and disinfectants.

The problem of vaginal discharges on breeder farms can be reduced by use of in-feed antibiotics and acidification products for the sow feeds. However, the high feed intake of sows means that the cost–benefit ratio to the farmer of this type of feed additive intervention needs to be assessed carefully.

1.11 Case Study

The farmer was the owner and operator of a large and complex farm system with breeder, nursery and finisher pig units on several farm sites. The farmer employed several farm managers to operate and manage parts of the breeding and farrowing farm areas, the separate weaner pig farm sites and the finishing pig farm sites. Several of these farm sites were in distant and isolated locations, for biosecurity reasons. A logistics and transport group moved the pigs on trucks on the roads between the various breeder farms, weaner farm sites and finisher sites. Over a period of months, the owner noticed that the number of finisher pigs sent on trucks to the market each week was consistently lower than target levels, when calculated from the breeder farm performance and projected number of finisher pigs. The owner then examined the breeder and production pig data supplied by the managers (Fig. 1.11i).

He calculated that on the main farm site of 500 sows, with normal mating and conception and farrowing rates, there should have been 20 litters born each week of the year, leading to a total of around 200 pigs weaned each week. The farmer inspected the breeder farm personally and confirmed that these sows were producing 20 litters per week, with 10 piglets weaned per litter and placed on to trucks for delivery to the weaner farms (Fig. 1.11ii). He then looked at the weaner and finisher pig data. While these production pigs had mild health problems, such as pneumonia and diarrhoea, these did not seem to be particularly severe. The production pig mortality charts for the pens indicated that the losses of pigs from the age of weaning until pigs were sent for slaughter, was at the target level of 5%. The days taken for these pigs to grow from weaning to slaughter age also seemed normal. The pigs stayed 6 weeks in the weaner areas and 11 weeks in the finisher areas. He therefore calculated that he should be sending around 190 pigs/week on to trucks to the slaughterhouse. However, when he looked at the records from his farm and the slaughterhouse, he noticed that for many weeks of the year, he sent only 180 pigs/week to slaughter.

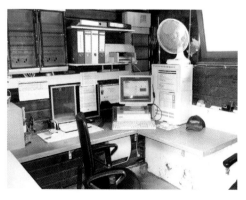

Fig. 1.11i. Tidy office of manager with pig farm data records.

Key Features

- The pigs seem normal.
- Production figures for one area of the pig farm are low.

1.11a. What is this problem?
1.11b. What are the important management systems required to prevent this problem?

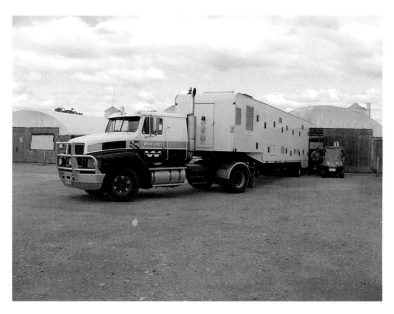

Fig. 1.11ii. Truck for transport of weaner pigs from breeder to production farm sites.

1.11 Comments

1.11a. This problem is probably the theft of weaner pigs, involving some of the farm managers and staff. Large and complex farm systems can have various problems with theft of pigs or pig feed or equipment, either by outside persons entering the farms, or by farm staff, or by groups that perform farm tasks on a contract basis. The vehicles of outside people entering the farm, such as electricians, can be searched. However, the theft of pigs or pig feed or equipment by farm staff or contractors can be difficult to detect. Some large farm systems will employ many diverse staff and managers, with contractor teams performing jobs such as pig transport, logistics, piglet processing, farm cleaning tasks, manure handling, building maintenance, etc. These teams may move frequently between various farm sites. The theft of pigs usually involves weaner pigs, as being relatively small they are easy to hide or transport in a private vehicle.

1.11b. Many farms will employ security personnel to guard against intruders and theft by outside persons. Prevention of thefts by farm staff or contractors requires vigilance by the farm owners and strategies to limit opportunities for bad practices to develop into problems. The farmer needs to continually evaluate herd performance by looking at farm data. Important data sets will include: (i) the percentage of pigs born that are sold; (ii) the number of pigs sold per sow per year; (iii) the number of post-weaning deaths; (iv) the number of days a batch of pigs requires to reach marketing weight; (v) the killing out or dressing percentage of the pigs at slaughter; (vi) the number of tonnes of feed supplied to the farm per sow; and (vii) the feed conversion ratio from wean to finish. Pig farms run best on a 52-week cycle – one batch of pigs/week. It usually takes a total of 21 weeks for a pig to move from its birth to final finisher pig weight. Farm workers must be free to report any suspicious activity by other farm staff or contract workers to managers.

1.12   Case Study

The farmer operated a small nursery and finisher pig farm, with groups of pigs kept in small older-style buildings and open-pasture pens. The farmer and his family also had a range of other farm livestock interests, such as goats and chickens, all moving around on the same farm site with the pigs. The farmer prepared home-mixed feeds for these live-stock. The chickens and pigs were raised in the same areas (Fig. 1.12i), with many wild birds also attracted to the open pens and feed. The nursery pigs were generally healthy and received a complete vaccination programme. The finisher pigs were alert and eating well, but some groups of pigs were considered to be uneven and slow in growth rates. The pig farmer was called by the operator of the local slaughterhouse, following the delivery of several finisher pigs from the farm. During the processing of these pigs, the slaughterhouse workers had noticed that the lymph nodes of pigs had some nodules. Close inspection indicated that the lymph nodes of the neck and jaw and those around the intestines of these pigs were enlarged and firm (Fig. 1.12ii). The surrounding tissues and the body organs of the pigs appeared relatively normal. When these lymph nodes were sectioned, the enlargement was found to be due to firm grey swelling, with some nodules of various sizes and yellow gritty areas within the nodules and swelling.

Key Features

- Pig farm production mixed with livestock and chickens.
- Firm grey swelling and nodules in the lymph nodes.

1.12a. What is this problem?
1.12b. What control measures may assist the herd?

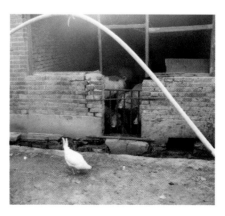

Fig. 1.12i. Pigs and chickens in small open farm.

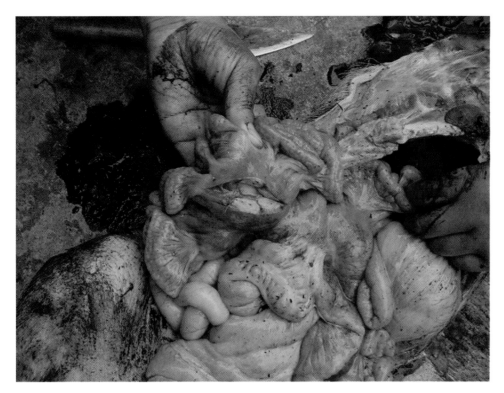

Fig. 1.12ii. Enlarged lymph nodes with grey nodular swelling.

1.12 Comments

1.12a. This problem is tuberculosis in pigs, due to infection with one of the *Mycobacterium* species. The Mycobacteria are a group of bacteria associated with the various forms of tuberculosis disease in cattle, goats, chickens, wild animals and humans. The types of Mycobacteria that affect pigs are usually the ones found in poultry and birds and from the environment, particularly the soil. The disease is not transmitted between pigs; each individual pig gains the bacterial infection from the environment or interaction with chickens. Tuberculosis in pigs is therefore usually seen in smaller farms where the pigs have prolonged access to soil, wildlife or chickens. On some farms, pigs may have access to chicken or wildlife carcass materials presented as feedstuffs. The bacteria are eaten by the pig and settle in the lymph nodes, causing the relatively minor lesions, seen at slaughter. Only rarely will pigs suffer a more severe clinical problem with this infection. In contrast to tuberculosis in cattle, the types of Mycobacteria and tuberculosis in pigs are not usually considered a threat to humans. The disease tuberculosis has a long history in humans and much of the examination of animals at slaughterhouses was aimed to detect these types of lesions, to prevent infected meat from entering the food chain.

1.12b. Infection of farm sites by tuberculosis will be reduced by removal of other livestock, such as chickens, poultry and wild animals from contact with pigs. Farmers preparing home-mixed feeds need to ensure all animal-material ingredients are properly sanitized and that storage areas do not allow carcasses to be placed among the feed ingredients.

PART 2
Deaths of Pigs in the Nursery Area

2.1   Case Study

The farmer operated a medium-sized farm system with breeder, nursery and finisher unit on a single large farm site. There were many other similar farms in the region. The farmer had purchased many gilts and boars and developed various new lines of modern pig breeds. The nursery and finisher pigs were raised in various new and older buildings. The performance of the breeder farm was poor, with a number of abortions noted and low numbers of pigs born alive. The farmer also noticed that over a period of 1 year the mortality rate among many of the groups of nursery pigs was high to very high (over 20%). Close inspection indicated that the weaner pig mortality started to increase in most of the groups between 4 and 10 weeks old. Many of these pigs were noticed to have some nasal discharges, sneezing and coughing. Occasionally, several pigs would die in a group in a 1 week period. Generally, the nursery pigs were dull and depressed with poor appetite. They were in poor body condition and were slow at getting to target weights. Many runt nursery pigs were noticed (Fig. 2.1i). At autopsy of the dead pigs, a wide range of problems was noted. In some pigs, there was a diffuse firmness and a mottled, tan colour to all the lobes of the lungs, including the front and rear lobes (Fig. 2.1ii). In some other pigs, there were also patchy areas of firm consolidation pneumonia, fibrin and pleurisy over some areas of the front lobes. The problems continued to persist for many months and did not respond to antibiotic and other medications.

Key Features

- High mortality and respiratory disease in nursery areas.
- Range of lung problems found in dead pigs at autopsy.

2.1a. What is this problem?
2.1b. What control measures may assist the herd?

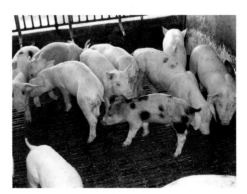

Fig. 2.1i. Groups of runt, dull and sick nursery pigs with some nasal discharges.

2.1 Comments

2.1a. This is the common respiratory disease and mortality situation in farms that have ongoing infections and problems with the porcine reproductive and respiratory syndrome (PRRS) virus. Many other virus and bacteria agents are also involved in the respiratory disease and deaths, so this problem is known as the porcine respiratory disease complex (PRDC). In this case study, the pigs were probably also infected with swine influenza virus, *Pasteurella* and *Mycoplasma* bacteria. The PRRS virus

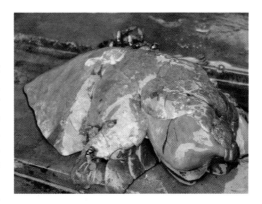

Fig. 2.1ii. Lung lesions in affected pig.

remains the number one health problem facing pigs around the world. The PRRS virus is carried in the wind and is easily inhaled by pigs from the excretions of infected pigs. It is infectious even in small doses and from all secretions of pigs (saliva, faeces, aerosol, semen). There is commonly cross-transmission between different age groups, such as from breeder pigs to nursery pigs. In nursery and grower pigs, it can cause a direct interstitial pneumonia; this is a type of pneumonia that attacks the blood vessels and linings of the airways in the lungs. Another part of the basis of the strong hold that PRRS has over pigs is its ability to attack and harm the macrophages in the lungs. These cells are the ones that normally roam around the surfaces of the lungs grabbing and killing viruses and bacteria that enter the lungs, when the pig takes in inspired air. So an outbreak of PRRS infections in a group of pigs can lead to this PRDC problem, with PRRS pneumonia and common secondary infections caused by these other viruses and bacteria. A farm that is active and positive for PRRS will commonly have a range of diseases and raised nursery mortality rates.

2.1b. The various secondary infections in PRDC, such as swine influenza, need to be considered for vaccination and medication programmes. The underlying PRRS virus has proved difficult to control, particularly in areas where there are many pig farms nearby and the virus can move around pig farms via aerosols in the wind. Because there are many strains, and new strains are continually evolving, then having a recent outbreak of PRRS does not provide any immunity to the next PRRS virus entry and disease outbreak. It is therefore a common and ongoing problem.

It has proved possible to eradicate PRRS infections from breeding farms, by operating a completely closed herd and waiting for immunity to develop in the sows. After some months, these immune sows can then be inseminated with PRRS-negative semen and produce PRRS-negative litters of piglets. These piglets may be raised to become PRRS-negative nursery and grower pigs, if they are also kept fully isolated from other pigs. For a farm system to use this process, requires good isolation of the farm sites and prevention of new infections in the future. It is therefore difficult to follow this programme in an area where there are many other pig farms nearby.

The control of PRRS therefore often relies on vaccines. Various PRRS vaccines are available. The modified live PRRS vaccines have been the most useful for providing protection. It is often important to establish what strain of PRRS virus is on the pig farm. This usually requires the use of PCR tests. For control of respiratory disease due to PRRS, the vaccine may be applied to piglets at 3 weeks old. However, current vaccines do not prevent infections with all PRRS strains and disease can still occur in vaccinated pigs.

2.2   Case Study

The farmer operated a breeder, nursery and finisher pig farm system, with modern lines of pig breeds. The breeder pigs and young piglets all received a complete vaccination programme. The weaned pigs were moved to the nursery production pig areas at 3–4 weeks old. The farmer also operated a feed-mixing and preparation facility on the same site, supplying all the different stages of feeds for the pigs. The feed components consisted of standard levels of cereals, soybeans and a vitamin and mineral supplement. The feed supplies were stored in open and exposed areas at the farm (Fig. 2.2i). The farmer noticed an increasing number of deaths of pigs in the late nursery stages, with several deaths over a period of weeks. Close inspection indicated that these deaths were always of the larger, rapidly growing pigs. The farm workers had invariably found these pigs dead, with no clinical signs noted. Many of the affected pigs were of Landrace breed but other pig breeds were also affected. The deaths were scattered among different pens in the nursery area, with the other pigs in these pens appearing normal. At autopsy of the dead pigs, the farmer and veterinarian noted that the heart was enlarged, with large splashy red haemorrhages and pale streaks throughout the heart muscle (Fig. 2.2.ii). There was a marked accumulation of soft pale jelly-like fluid in the sac around the heart and in the lungs.

Key Features

- Scattered deaths among large, rapidly growing nursery pigs.
- Splash haemorrhages across the heart and excess fluid in the sac around the heart.

2.2a. What is this problem?
2.2b. What control measures may assist the herd?

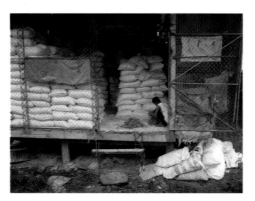

Fig. 2.2i. Open pig-feed storage areas.

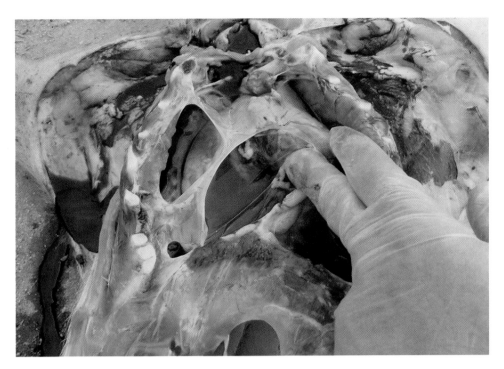

Fig. 2.2ii. Fluid in the sac around the heart and haemorrhages across heart muscle.

2.2 Comments

2.2a. This is a specific condition in pigs known as mulberry heart disease. It is a common problem on many pig farms around the world. It is not an infectious disease, but is caused by a deficiency in the diet of vitamin E and selenium. These vitamins are necessary for maintaining the integrity of blood vessels in the body, so a deficiency will lead to leaky blood vessels. In the pig, this develops in the heart of the rapidly growing pig, with haemorrhages and loss of heart function, causing sudden death. Vitamin E is a fat-based vitamin and is delivered to the baby piglet via colostrum. After weaning from the sow, pigs experience a drop in the levels of vitamin E in their blood and tissues. This vitamin must therefore be supplied in adequate levels in the fat components of the pig diet after weaning. A common feature of many farm problems with vitamin E deficiency and mulberry heart disease is the poor storage of prepared feed. Vitamin E (and other vitamins) will decay during feed storage, and will decay more rapidly if the feed is stored in hot areas.

2.2b. When cases of mulberry heart disease are diagnosed on a pig farm, it is often necessary to inject the groups of weaner pigs with vitamin E and selenium. It may also require further addition of these components in the feed supply. The levels of vitamin E in the diet, which were stated to be adequate in some older textbooks or nutrition handbooks, have not proven to be sufficient for modern lines of larger pig breeds, such as Landrace. A current suggested diet level for weaner pigs would be 250 IU (international units)/kg of prepared feed. Selenium levels in pig diets are usually limited to 0.3 ppm.

2.3 Case Study

The farmer operated a medium-sized breeder and nursery and finisher farm, with modern lines of pig breeds. The farrowing rates and numbers of piglets born alive were at the target levels. The farmer used a complete vaccination programme for the breeding pigs. The farm was located in an area with many other farms in the region. Trucks moved between these farms for feed delivery and collection of dead pigs and dead piglets. There was an ongoing outbreak of yellow diarrhoea and vomiting among numerous litters of 2–4-week-old piglets in the farrowing areas. The weaned pigs were moved to the nursery production pig areas at 3–4 weeks old. The farmer noticed that the nursery areas experienced a high level of mortality, with numerous weaner pigs with diarrhoea and many deaths. Close inspection indicated that affected weaner pigs had large amounts of yellow to green to brown diarrhoea faeces (Fig. 2.3i). These pigs were dull and not eating well. The affected pigs did not respond to antibiotic treatments and many pigs became runted and weak (Fig. 2.3ii). At autopsy of sick pigs, the farmer and veterinarian noticed that the small intestines were distended with watery, yellow fluid. The mucosal lining of the intestines appeared thin.

Key Features

- Yellow to green to brown diarrhoea in weaner pigs.
- High rates of mortality in young weaner pigs.

2.3a. What is this problem?
2.3b. What control measures may assist the herd?

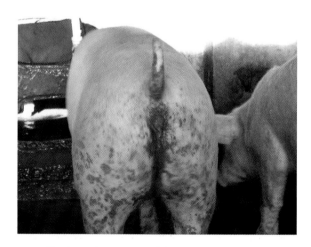

Fig. 2.3i. Yellow–green diarrhoea in weaner piglets.

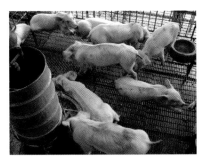

Fig. 2.3ii. Groups of runt weaner piglets in poor condition.

2.3 Comments

2.3a. This type of high mortality and multi-coloured (rainbow) diarrhoea cases in weaner pigs is the common current form of porcine epidemic diarrhoea (PED). It is usually seen in conjunction with diarrhoea cases in baby piglets (see Case Study 5.6). PED is caused by a pig coronavirus. There are a group of related coronaviruses in pigs around the world, which cause very similar forms of this disease, including viruses known as transmissible gastroenteritis (TGE) and haemagglutinating encephalitis virus (HEV). At the moment, PED is the most common and important form of pig coronavirus disease, with recent spread around many pig farming regions in Asia and globally. Outbreaks of PED vary in intensity and duration, sometimes with many older pigs affected also. The outbreaks are often worse on farms that are also positive for American strains of PRRS. The diagnosis of PED can be confirmed by blood tests or PCR tests. In some farms, new PED outbreaks can recur in young piglets every 6–12 months.

2.3b. Young sick pigs may be fed with high-energy soft feed products and provided with warmth while they are nursed to recovery. The treatment of diarrhoea pigs may also be to provide rehydration electrolytes. These electrolytes may be given by a clean syringe into the mouth or rectum of each young pig.

The main method for limiting the duration of an outbreak of PED remains the use of controlled exposure of the breeder pigs to live PED virus-positive material, derived from fresh, affected piglet intestines. Control of outbreaks on problem farms remains largely an attempt to raise herd immunity by use of this live-virus feedback material. This acts to enhance natural immunity of the breeder herd and increase maternal antibodies in the sow colostrum, so providing some protection to the young piglets. The most successful programmes are therefore usually when the sows and gilts are exposed several times to the feedback material. Exposing the sows and gilts may also result in depression, apathy and anorexia and abortions.

A number of local attenuated and killed vaccines for PED are available. The actual usefulness of these various PED vaccines on problem farms has probably been very limited. This may be due to virus factors such as the fact that PED is a small RNA virus with a strong ability to mutate, creating new strains on farms that may be resistant to vaccine strains.

The control of PED on farms also requires reduction of rodent and bird populations and restriction of their entry to farms and feed areas. Great care and attention must be paid to cleaning any trucks that enter the farm, particularly those that may be carrying or collecting live or dead pigs.

2.4   Case Study

The farmer operated a breeder, nursery and finisher pig farm system, with modern lines of pig breeds in several medium-sized breeder herds. The breeder pigs and young piglets all received a complete vaccination programme. The weaned pigs were moved in some older trucks to the separate and distant nursery production pig areas at 3–4 weeks old. There was some mixing of batches from different breeder farm origins. The mortality rate in the initial post-weaning phase increased after addition of the weaner pigs arriving from a new breeding herd into this system. Close inspection indicated that the mortality figures for the pigs between 3 and 10 weeks old had increased greatly. The hospital pens of the nursery sites also contained many sick and dull pigs (Fig. 2.4i), but there was no clear pattern of diarrhoea or coughing in these pigs. These groups of weaner pigs had many smaller runt pigs, which were dull and did not eat properly and struggled to gain weight through the weaner and later grower-pig phases. At autopsy of affected weaner pigs, the farmer and veterinarian noticed these pigs had a dull pale thickening in patchy strands and sheets across the linings of the lungs, heart and abdominal organs, such as the liver. In some pigs, this patchy grey–yellow thickening of the linings around the lungs and heart sac was thicker and resembled two pieces of bread and butter stuck together (Fig. 2.4ii).

Key Features

- Mixed sources of weaned pigs into the farm nursery.
- Mortality and runt pigs in the nursery period of 5–10 weeks old.
- Distinctive patchy thickening of the serosa over the linings of the heart, lungs and liver.

2.4a. What is this problem?
2.4b. What control measures may assist the herd?

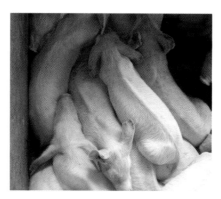

Fig. 2.4i. Numerous cases of illness and deaths among weaner piglets.

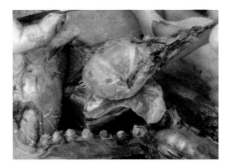

Fig. 2.4ii. Thickening of the linings of the heart sac and lungs.

2.4 Comments

2.4a. The signs are consistent with diffuse inflammation of the body linings (known as serositis) in pigs caused by the bacterium *Haemophilus parasuis* (HPS). This disease is also often known as Glasser's disease. It is a common disease of pig farms around the world. Pigs are usually affected in the period soon after weaning, but the nasty disease lesions can linger and be visible in or around the lungs and heart of older pigs. The pigs on most farms have a stable flora of strains of HPS in their throats, but these strains vary from farm to farm. Piglets in stable herds are usually infected within a few days of birth from their mother and develop a sub-clinical infection and acquire protective immunity. However, in situations like this case study, where piglets are mixed with piglets from other breeder farms, which may have different strains of HPS, then all the piglets will lack appropriate maternal antibody. The bacteria will not encounter any resistance and many of the young weaned pigs will develop Glasser's disease. It can be difficult to confirm the diagnosis by culture of the HPS bacterium from Glasser's disease cases. Some points to improve success include: (i) taking the culture from freshly sick animals, importantly from pigs that have not yet been specifically medicated for the disease; and (ii) ensuring that the laboratory has experience at culturing this difficult bacterium.

2.4b. The response of groups of pigs with Glasser's disease to antibiotic medication is often fairly weak. Pigs that have already become runted will often show little response. Appropriate staffing levels to handle feeding, nursing and treatment programmes are needed. Attention to the warm temperature and low draught requirements of these pigs is important. Some vaccines are available for Glasser's disease, but these may only cover a few strains of the bacterium, and so are limited in their usefulness on many farms.

Use of in-feed antibiotic therapy to control the spread of Glasser's disease in weaner pigs during the post-weaning phase is currently an essential part of pig farming. This form of control has the advantages of not requiring detailed knowledge of maternal antibody status, nor of the dominant strains of HPS present on the affected farm. HPS isolates often show full sensitivity to florfenicol and amoxicillin. Reliable in-feed or in-water medications are preferred for Glasser's disease control, as the use of injectable products will lead to gaps in suitable blood concentrations over the post-weaning period when the agent may be circulating in the blood of infected pigs. Any relaxation of the antibiotic medication, once started, is likely to lead to a fresh rise in cases.

2.5   Case Study

The farmer operated an established breeder, nursery and finisher pig farm system. There were many smaller pig farms in the region and some of the farm workers kept pigs in their backyard settings at home. The farmer also occasionally purchased various sows and nursery pigs from these local farms. The farmer had experienced a range of disease problems, therefore used a lot of pig treatments, but he was concerned about farm costs and did not use many commercial vaccines. The feed for the pigs was derived from various local sources, including by-products and food waste. The farmer noticed an increase in mortality and illness in the pigs in the nursery areas – up to 20% mortality over a period of several weeks. Close inspection indicated that the dead and dying weaner pigs had a dark congestion and blackened colour to their ears and snouts, known as cyanosis (Fig. 2.5i). Many of the sick pigs were dull and listless. Pigs seemed to slowly wander around in an aimless manner – the pig has nowhere to go and is in no hurry to get there. The pigs tended to lie down and huddle in piles. Many pigs also had sticky dark discharges noticeable at their eyes. Some pigs appeared to have yellow diarrhoea and some were vomiting yellow fluids. At autopsy of the dead pigs, bloody haemorrhages were noticed in many of the lymph nodes and inside the urinary bladder. The kidneys seemed pale, with many small bloody spots on the surface (Fig. 2.5ii). The spleen was a normal size but had some rough dark areas at the edges. Blood tests showed that the pigs had a low white blood cell count (leukopenia). The pigs did not respond to antibiotic therapy treatments.

Key Features

- High mortality rates in groups of nursery pigs.
- Conjunctivitis and haemorrhages in lymph nodes in affected pigs.

2.5a. What is this problem?
2.5b. What control measures may assist the herd?

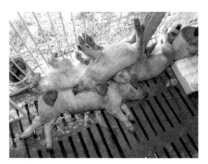

Fig. 2.5i. Numerous dead and dying weaner pigs with cyanosis.

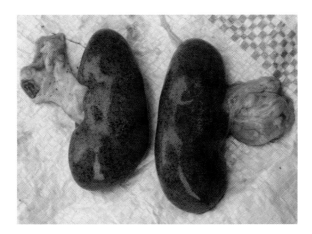

Fig. 2.5ii. Pale spotty kidneys and bladder haemorrhage.

2.5 Comments

2.5a. The high mortality and the autopsy signs are suggestive of classical swine fever (CSF), which is caused by a pestivirus. CSF is also known as hog cholera in some countries. The case study illustrates CSF on a farm with variable levels of immunity, where many weaner pigs are susceptible to the virus and many deaths occur. CSF is often known as a 'great imitator' and the clinical signs in the sick pigs are often vague or inconclusive and may resemble other diseases. CSF can be confirmed by blood tests and virus tests such as PCR.

2.5b. Affected pigs do not respond well to antibiotics or other treatments. A vaccination programme must be implemented for farms that are positive for CSF. Commercial vaccines exist for CSF in many regions. A course of different CSF vaccines from international suppliers, such as the live attenuated C strain and the subunit E2 vaccines, should be implemented. However, full protection against this disease in farms located in endemic and high-risk pig farming areas can be difficult, even with these vaccination programmes. This is because the disease is very common and pigs may be exposed early in life, so the vaccine administration may actually occur at around the same time as the pigs are exposed to wild 'hot' virus and while there is still some interference to protection from maternal antibodies. On many farms in this situation, it is therefore often necessary to develop multiple vaccine points around the time of weaning and early grower period.

The general effort required to keep diseases out, or to manage their entry in a practical manner, is known as external biosecurity. The various factors in the effort to keep out CSF are: (i) consideration of the purchase of replacement pigs and semen, to ensure that they are from reliable, disease-free sources; (ii) the control of staff and visitors; and (iii) control over the entry of pigs, vehicles, equipment and pork product on to farms. In this case study, it is possible that farm workers may have introduced the infection on to the larger farm from their backyard pigs, via boots, clothing or perhaps pork products. It is vital that all pork products are excluded from pig farm areas, including canteens. It is important not to allow farm workers or visitors to provide any outside food waste to farm pigs.

2.6 Case Study

The farmer operated an established medium-sized breeder, nursery and finisher farm system. There had been many different sources of pigs to the farm over the years, with various age groups and breeds now present on the farm. The farmer had experienced a range of disease problems, therefore used a lot of pig treatments, but he was concerned about farm costs and did not use many commercial vaccines. The farmer noticed an increasing and serious problem with poor condition and stunting in pigs through the nursery and early grower stages (Fig. 2.6i). Close inspection indicated that many of these pigs showed rough hair coats, very poor growth rates, with many runt pigs. There were occasional cases of harsh breathing, occasional cases of diarrhoea, but no consistent clinical pattern. The hospital pens in the nursery had many sick pigs, which did not recover and died. In most batches, the problems seemed to be in pigs at 4–10 weeks old, with 10–20% of the batches affected. In occasional cases, the pigs had a yellow to orange colour to their body (jaundice). At autopsy of many pigs, the farmer and veterinarian noticed that the pigs were in poor body condition, with depletion of fat reserves, and some inflammation of the liver, colon and kidney. In particular, they noticed that lymph nodes around the body were greatly enlarged. This was most noticeable in the abdominal lymph nodes and the nodes in the inguinal region (Fig. 2.6ii).

Key Features

- Wasting pigs with poor performance in weaner and grower pigs.
- Range of diarrhoea, jaundice and coughing signs in some pigs.
- Enlarged lymph nodes in the abdomen and inguinal region.

2.6a. What is this problem?
2.6b. What control measures may assist the herd?

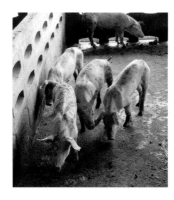

Fig. 2.6i. Sick and runt weaner pigs with very poor growth rates.

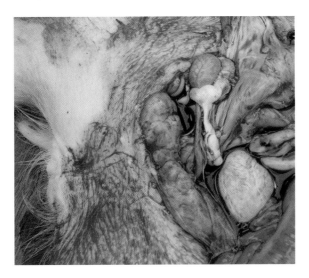

Fig. 2.6ii. Autopsy with enlarged inguinal lymph nodes.

2.6 Comments

2.6a. This is post-weaning multi-systemic wasting syndrome (PMWS) and enlarged lymph nodes, caused by active infections of pigs with porcine circovirus 2 (PCV-2). Many of the affected weaner pigs do not recover and the mortality rates in older weaner pigs can be very high. PCV-2 is a very common infection of pigs affecting farms all over the world. When this PCV-2 infection rises to a high level of virus in the blood and tissues, the damaging effects of the PCV-2 on lymph nodes and other tissues develop fully and the clinical signs occur. PCV-2 has several damaging effects on pigs. It has a direct effect on lymph nodes, causing damage, necrosis and enlargement. This is connected with a strong immune-suppressive effect, causing a general reduction in the pig's ability to fight secondary infections. During the many years when this disease and its aetiological agent were not clearly recognized, many nursery and grower pigs were affected, many farms lost profitability and the problem was designated as PMWS. A large number of treatments were tried with little success. The development of effective vaccines has led to a dramatic reduction in the incidence of this wasting problem.

2.6b. The thin weaner pigs do not respond well to antibiotics or other treatments and generally should be culled. PCV-2 infection and its associated disease issues have been dramatically brought under control in pig populations in the past 10 years, by the introduction of effective commercial vaccines.

All farmers are urged to add PCV-2 vaccines to their vaccine list, as they are highly beneficial to the profitability of pig farming, when applied to the pigs in a proper manner. The sick pigs presented in this case study farm are therefore due to the farmer failing to use PCV-2 vaccines in a proper manner.

The main factors that cause PCV-2 infections to develop to a high level in some pigs are now considered to be the presence of co-infections (such as the common pig viruses, PRRS or parvovirus) and the pigs being of a susceptible breed, such as Landrace.

2.7   Case Study

The farmer operated an established farm system with various breeder, nursery and finisher units on different sites. The breeder pigs and young piglets all received a complete vaccination programme. The breeding farm had a successful programme of modern genetics, with different farm sites having a variety of modern pig breeds. The weaned pigs from the different breeder farm areas were moved to a single nursery production pig area at 3–4 weeks old. There was a noticeable increase in the mortality of the current groups of nursery-stage pigs, compared with the previous 3 months (Fig. 2.7i). A similar surge in mortality levels had been noted around 6–12 months previously. Close inspection indicated that affected pigs were 5–10 weeks old; they were seen to be dull and separate from the group. These pigs did not eat well and often did not recover, became recumbent and died. At autopsy of some of the affected pigs, the farmer and veterinarian noticed there were fine strands of inflammatory material (fibrin) across the liver and other abdominal organs (Fig. 2.7ii), with an excess amount of pale cloudy fluid in the abdominal and chest cavities.

Key Features

- Mortality in nursery-age pigs.
- Many affected pigs with inflammation of body organ linings (serositis).

2.7a. What is this problem?
2.7b. What control measures may assist the herd?

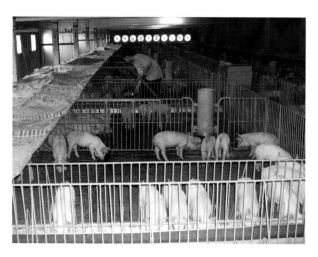

Fig. 2.7i. Weaner groups with high mortality.

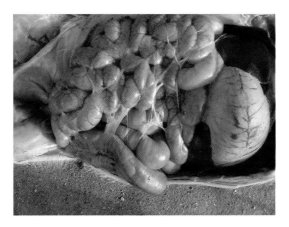
Fig. 2.7ii. Fine strands of fibrin across the body organ linings.

2.7 Comments

2.7a. These cases are pigs affected with bacterial blood poisoning (known as septicaemia) caused by the bacterium *Streptococcus suis*, which is a common bacterial infection in pigs. This bacterium lives in the environment of pig farms in dust and faeces in sheds and in carrier pigs. The clinical disease may include mortality, nervous signs and joint infections and is common on many farms around the world, typically in a proportion of pigs some weeks after weaning. The problem tends to occur in sporadic outbreaks and can reappear after some change in management or medication programmes. The bacterium enters the bloodstream of some pigs and often settles in the brain or joints, causing nervous convulsions and deaths. However, as in this case study, the main presenting sign can be a raised mortality rate in the weaner pigs, with few specific signs. The *S. suis* bacterium can be cultured from the organs of affected pigs if samples from an untreated pig are submitted to a bacteriology laboratory, to confirm the diagnosis of streptococcal septicaemia.

Infection in human pig-farm workers can occur when the dead pigs in this situation are subject to autopsy or dissection by workers who transfer blood from the affected pig into their own bloodstream, via unskilled knife cuts. Outbreaks and incidents of streptococcal infections in humans from this source occur globally, but have been more prominent in areas with weaker regulations or knowledge surrounding disposal and consumption of farm pigs.

2.7b. Pigs affected in an outbreak situation can be given injections of a penicillin antibiotic and placed into a quiet hospital-pen area. Some of these treated pigs can recover well.

There are no current vaccines that are effective for *S. suis*. Therefore strategic medication of weaner pigs is often needed to prevent damaging problems. In-feed or in-water penicillin antibiotics are the most effective for this weaner medication programme.

The occurrence of streptococcal infections is often associated with mixing of weaner pigs from different sources. Therefore the development of farm management systems that streamline groups of weaner pigs from one breeder-farm source into a single nursery pig flow, with all-in, all-out management can generally reduce the number of cases of this common disease.

2.8 Case Study

The farmer operated a medium-sized farm system with breeder farms and nursery and finisher sites at separate locations. The weaned pigs were moved in trucks on to the nursery sites from the breeder farms, with some mixing of batches from different farm origins. There were many other similar pig farms in the region. The performance of the breeder farms was poor, with a number of abortions noted and low numbers of pigs born alive. The farmer also noticed over a period of 1 year that the mortality rate among many of the groups of nursery pigs was high to very high (sometimes over 20%). Close inspection indicated that the weaner mortality started to increase in most of the groups between 4 and 10 weeks old. There was a general increase in the incidence of lethargy, coughing and harsh breathing among these pigs. These groups of weaner pigs had many smaller runt pigs (Fig. 2.8i), which were dull and did not eat properly and struggled to gain weight through the grower-pig phases. The hospital pens of the nursery site contained many sick and dull pigs. At autopsy of affected weaner pigs, the farmer and veterinarian noticed these pigs had well-demarcated, consolidated purple–red–grey areas in the front lobes of the lungs. There were some areas of pale yellow pus in occasional areas of these consolidated lobes. There was also some pleurisy and thickening of the surface of these areas of the lungs, with a dull, pale thickening in patchy strands and sheets across the linings of the lungs, heart and abdominal organs, such as the liver and intestines (Fig. 2.8ii). In some pigs, this patchy grey–yellow thickening of the linings around the lungs and heart sac was thicker and butter-like.

Key Features

- Mixed sources of weaned pigs into the farm nursery.
- High incidence of mortality and runt pigs at 4–10 weeks old.
- Distinctive patchy thickening of the serosa over the linings of the heart, lungs and liver.

2.8a. What is this problem?
2.8b. What control measures may assist the herd?

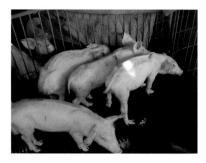

Fig. 2.8i. Numerous runt pigs and deaths among weaner piglets.

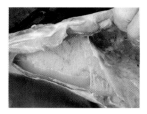

Fig. 2.8ii. Thickening of the linings of the abdomen, lungs and heart sac.

2.8 Comments

2.8a. This is a general nursery mortality disease situation due to ongoing infections and problems with the PRRS virus, combined in particular with diffuse inflammation of the body linings (known as serositis) in pigs caused by the bacterium *Haemophilus parasuis* (HPS). This situation is therefore a combination problem of PRRS with HPS. This is a common problem causing high levels of weaner pig mortality on pig farms around the world. It is often noticed in situations where weaner pigs are mixed with pigs from various breeder farms. The disease caused by HPS is also known as Glasser's disease.

The PRRS virus is also a common infection in pigs around the world and has many strains. The PRRS virus is carried in the wind and is easily inhaled by pigs from the excretions of infected pigs. It is infectious even in small doses and from all secretions of pigs (saliva, faeces, aerosol, semen). There is commonly cross-transmission between different age groups, such as from breeder pigs to nursery pigs. In nursery and grower pigs, PRRS infections in a group of pigs can have many consequences for the respiratory system. This will include the diffuse pneumonia and also common secondary infections by other bacteria, such as HPS. So a farm with PRRS infections will commonly have a range of diseases and raised mortality rates.

2.8b. The response of groups of pigs with PRRS and Glasser's disease to antibiotic medication is often weak. Pigs that have already become runted will often show little response. Appropriate staffing levels to handle feeding, nursing and treatment programmes are needed. Attention to the warm temperature and low draught requirements of these pigs is important. Some vaccines are available for Glasser's disease, but these may only cover a few strains of the bacterium, and so are limited in their usefulness on many farms. Use of in-feed antibiotic therapy or in-water medications to control the spread of Glasser's disease in weaner pigs during the post-weaning phase is currently an essential part of pig farming. HPS isolates often show full sensitivity to florfenicol and amoxicillin.

PRRS virus has proved difficult to control, particularly in areas where there are many pig farms in nearby areas and the virus can move around pig farms via aerosols in the wind. Because there are many strains, and new strains are continually evolving, then having a recent outbreak of PRRS does not provide any immunity to the next PRRS virus entry and disease outbreak. It is therefore a common and ongoing problem. The attempted control of PRRS in areas with many pig farms often relies on vaccines. Various PRRS vaccines are available. The modified live PRRS vaccines have been useful at providing some protection to pigs, which may be exposed to PRRS virus strains similar to the ones present in the vaccine. It is often important to establish what strain of PRRS virus is on the pig farm. For control of respiratory disease due to PRRS, the vaccine may be applied to piglets at 3 weeks old. However, current vaccines do not prevent infections with all PRRS strains and disease can still occur in vaccinated pigs.

2.9 Case Study

The farmer operated a newly organized breeder, nursery and finisher pig farm system, with modern lines of pig breeds. The breeder pigs and young piglets all received a complete vaccination programme. The weaned pigs were moved to the separate nursery production pig areas at 3–4 weeks old. The breeders and weaners appeared to be stable for the PRRS virus. The mortality rate in the post-weaning phase at the nursery site appeared to have increased slightly over a period of weeks. Close inspection of the mortality figures of the pigs between 5 and 10 weeks old confirmed a moderate increase in pig deaths, with the hospital pens of the nursery site containing several sick and dull pigs. These pigs seemed to have some chest pain and breathed and stretched in an altered manner, when they were disturbed. There was no clear pattern of diarrhoea or coughing in these pigs. These groups of weaner pigs had some smaller runt pigs, which were dull and did not eat properly and struggled to gain weight through the weaner and later grower-pig phases (Fig. 2.9i). At autopsy of affected weaner pigs, the farmer and veterinarian noticed these pigs had a dull, pale thickening in patchy strands and sheets across the linings of the lungs, heart and abdominal organs, such as the liver (Fig. 2.9ii). Samples were sent from these pigs to a local bacteriology laboratory, but no specific bacteria were cultured.

Key Features

- Mortality and runt pigs in the nursery period of 5–10 weeks old.
- Patchy thickening of the serosa over the linings of the heart, lungs and liver.

2.9a. What is this problem?
2.9b. What control measures may assist the herd?

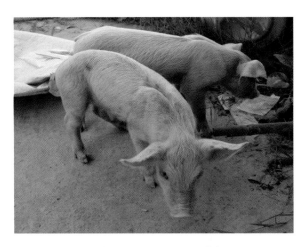

Fig. 2.9i. Occasional runts and deaths among weaner piglets.

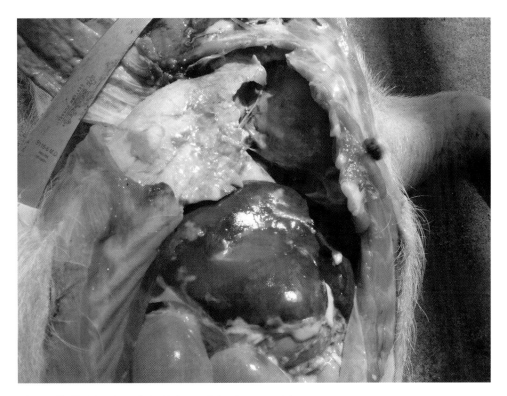

Fig. 2.9ii. Thickening of the linings of the lungs and heart sac.

2.9 Comments

2.9a. The sign of diffuse inflammation of the body linings (known as serositis) in pigs can be suggestive of disease caused by the small bacterium *Mycoplasma hyorhinis*. This disease is not considered common, but does occur occasionally in some modern pig farms. The signs in pigs are similar but milder than those seen with Glasser's disease, so it can be important to pursue further diagnostic tests, such as PCR, to clarify the cause of these problems. *M. hyorhinis* is a separate bacterial species to the more common *Mycoplasma hyopneumoniae*, which causes enzootic pneumonia with coughing and to *Mycoplasma hyosynoviae*, which causes joint infections and lameness. *M. hyorhinis* lives in the nasal cavity of many normal pigs.

2.9b. Groups of affected pigs may be placed into warm, well-ventilated areas and treated with appropriate antibiotics, such as tylosin, tiamulin or lincomycin. It is also possible to place strategic medication into the feed or water for groups of pigs likely to be in danger of this disease, such as when pigs are mixed and grouped together.

There are no vaccines for *M. hyorhinis*, and the vaccines for the enzootic pneumonia agent *M. hyopneumoniae* do not work against this agent. The immunity of most herds to this agent probably builds up over time, and the number of cases in any new herd will diminish once herd immunity develops fully.

2.10 Case Study

The farmer operated a large breeder, nursery and finisher farm system, in a region with many other pig farms. The farm site had a variety of buildings for each phase of production. The breeder pigs and young piglets received an intermittent vaccination programme. The farmer sometimes purchased weaner and breeder pigs from other nearby farms and placed them into the herd to increase production numbers. The farmer noticed many depressed pigs and an increase in mortality in the nursery areas. Close inspection indicated that many pigs in most of the nursery and grower farm buildings had become sick, dull and depressed, particularly the younger nursery pigs. The farmer commented that it appeared that the whole nursery-farm area had stopped. Many of the sick weaner pigs at 3–9 weeks old showed some intermittent sneezing, with eye and nasal discharges and some coughing (Fig. 2.10i). Some of the older pigs, 10–15 weeks old were also sick and seemed to be wobbling when they walked. At autopsy of the weaner pigs, the farmer and veterinarian noticed that there was some speckled white areas of necrosis of the tonsils and larynx area in the throat of some pigs, and some inflammation of the nasal cavity of some pigs (Fig. 2.10ii), but few other signs.

Key Features

- Farm in pig-dense area.
- Many sick pigs in weaner group with sneezing, eye and nasal discharges.

2.10a. What is this problem?
2.10b. What control measures may assist the herd?

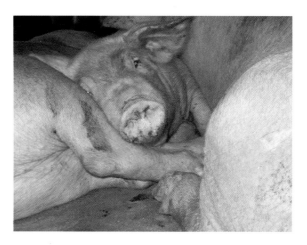

Fig. 2.10i. Sick weaner pigs with sneezing and nasal discharges.

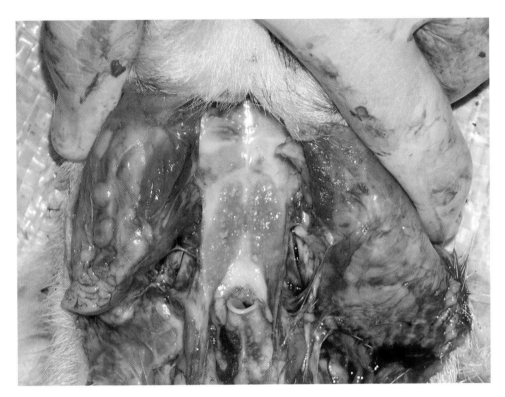

Fig. 2.10ii. Autopsy of weaner pig with inflammation of the tonsils and nasal cavity.

2.10 Comments

2.10a. This type of herd problem with sick weaner pigs and upper respiratory tract signs in nursery pigs is suggestive of pseudorabies. This disease is due to a pig herpes virus and is also known as Aujesky's disease in some countries. Outbreaks of disease are now less common, because of the widespread availability of useful vaccines and eradication programmes in some countries. However, in regions that remain positive for pseudorabies, it is a common disease of pigs, particularly in larger herds. It is often seen as a background problem on many farms, with occasional outbreaks of more severe illness and mortality. The virus is easily spread via pig to pig contact, so farms experience infections where new pigs are introduced. In some pig farm areas, boars may be shared between farms, or farms may purchase many pigs, as in this case study. When a pig is infected, the virus develops in the throat and spreads to the lungs. It can also travel from the throat via the nerves into the brain, causing nervous signs, which are more likely to be seen in older pigs.

2.10b. Pseudorabies is generally controlled by the use of modern commercial vaccines. During an outbreak, the herd should be vaccinated and sick animals removed. This will lead to a recovery of the herd and may even eliminate the problem in the herd. There are various types of vaccines available, which can be given routinely to pigs in an infected herd. The repeated use of vaccines over some years can lead to full herd protection and elimination of clinical problems in small herds. However, in larger herds (more than 200 sows) the vaccines do not eliminate the disease, even when used for long periods.

2.11   Case Study

The farmer operated a medium-sized farm system with breeder, nursery and finisher unit on a single large-farm site. There were many other similar farms in the region. The farmer had purchased many gilts and boars and developed various new lines of modern pig breeds. The nursery and finisher pigs were raised in various new and older buildings. The performance of the breeder farm was poor, with a number of abortions noted and low numbers of pigs born alive. The farmer also noticed that over a period of 1 year the mortality rate among many of the groups of nursery pigs was high to very high (sometimes over 20%). Close inspection indicated that this mortality started to increase in most of the groups between 4 and 10 weeks old. Many of these pigs were noticed to have some nasal discharges, sneezing and many also had deep persistent coughing. Generally, the nursery pigs were dull and depressed with poor appetite (Fig. 2.11i). They were in poor body condition and were slow at getting to target weights. At autopsy of the dead pigs, a wide range of problems was noted. In some pigs, there was a diffuse firmness and a mottled, tan colour to all the lobes of the lungs, including the front and rear lobes (Fig. 2.11ii). In some other pigs, there were also patchy areas of firm consolidation pneumonia, fibrin and pleurisy over some areas of the front lobes and inflammation of the linings of the heart sac. In some other pigs, there was inflammation of the lining of the abdomen, known as peritonitis. The problems continued to persist for many months and did not respond to antibiotic and other medications.

Key Features

- High mortality and respiratory disease in nursery areas.
- Range of lung problems found in dead pigs at autopsy.

2.11a. What is this problem?
2.11b. What control measures may assist the herd?

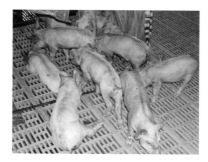

Fig. 2.11i. Groups of runt, dull, sick and coughing nursery pigs.

2.11 Comments

2.11a. This is the common respiratory disease and mortality situation in farms that have ongoing infections and problems with the PRRS virus. Many other viruses and bacteria are also involved in respiratory disease and deaths, so this problem is known as PRDC. In this case study, the pigs were also probably infected with swine influenza virus and bacteria such as *Haemophilus*

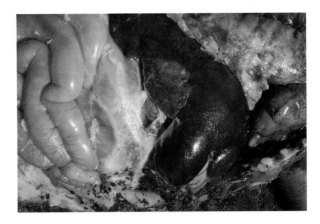

Fig. 2.11ii. Peritonitis and lung lesions in affected pigs.

parasuis, *Pasteurella*, *Streptococcus* and *Mycoplasma*. The PRRS virus is infectious even in small doses and from all secretions of pigs (saliva, faeces, aerosol, semen). There is commonly cross-transmission between different age groups, such as from breeder pigs to nursery pigs. Another part of the basis of the strong hold that PRRS has over pigs is its ability to attack and harm the macrophages in the lungs. These cells are the ones that normally roam around the surfaces of the lungs grabbing and killing viruses and bacteria that enter the lungs, when the pig takes in inspired air. So an outbreak of PRRS infections in a group of pigs can often lead to this PRDC problem, with the PRRS pneumonia and common secondary infections caused by these other viruses and bacteria. So a farm with PRRS infections will commonly have a range of diseases and raised mortality rates in the nursery area. In some farm situations, where other major infections such as CSF also occur then mortality in the nursery area can reach very high levels of 20–30%.

2.11b. The various secondary infections in PRDC need to be considered for vaccination and medication programmes. The underlying PRRS virus has proved difficult to control, particularly in areas where there are many pig farms in nearby areas. Because there are many strains, and new strains are continually evolving, then having a recent outbreak of PRRS does not provide any immunity to the next PRRS virus entry and disease outbreak. It is therefore a common and ongoing problem.

It has proved possible to eradicate PRRS infections from some breeding farms, by operating a completely closed herd and waiting for immunity to develop in the sows. After some months, these immune sows can then be inseminated with PRRS-negative semen and produce PRRS-negative litters of piglets. These piglets may be raised to become PRRS-negative nursery and grower pigs, if they are also kept fully isolated from other pigs. For a farm system to use this process requires good isolation of the farm sites and prevention of new infections in the future. It is therefore difficult to follow this programme in an area with many other pig farms nearby.

The control of PRRS therefore often relies on vaccines. Various PRRS vaccines are available. The modified live PRRS vaccines have been useful at providing some protection to pigs, which may be exposed to PRRS virus strains similar to the ones present in the vaccine. It is often important to establish what strain of PRRS virus is on the pig farm. This usually requires the use of PCR tests. For control of respiratory disease complex due to PRRS, the vaccine may be applied to piglets at 3 weeks old. However, current vaccines do not prevent infections with all PRRS strains and disease can still occur in vaccinated pigs.

PART 3
Deaths of Finisher and Older Pigs

3.1 Case Study

The farmer operated a medium-sized breeder, nursery and finisher farm system. There were many smaller pig farms in the region. The farmer occasionally purchased various sows and nursery pigs from these local farms. The breeder pigs and young piglets all received a complete vaccination programme. The feed for the pigs was derived from various local sources, including local by-products and food waste. Groups of finisher pigs were sold to local markets, when they reached slaughter weight. The farmer was concerned by an outbreak of numerous deaths, which occurred among all the various groups of farm pigs, with rapid illness and death. The sick and dead pigs had red haemorrhagic patches on the skin over their bodies. Close inspection indicated that the affected sick pigs became dull, sick and huddled together. The skin of these pigs became congested, red and purple over the ears and snout (known as cyanosis). There was no response to antibiotics or other treatments in any of the pigs. After 2 or 3 days of being ill, the sick pigs collapsed and died (Fig. 3.1i). Very few pigs recovered, with large numbers of dead pigs of various ages piling up in the walkways and pits of the farm. At autopsy of these pigs, the farmer and veterinarian noticed bloody congestion, oedema fluid swelling and haemorrhages through the body, including the kidney and the enlarged lymph nodes. The spleen was also greatly enlarged and filled with blood (Fig. 3.1ii).

Key Features

- Rapid spread and high death rates in all pigs, including adults.
- Pigs with cyanosis, haemorrhagic lymph nodes, kidney and spleen.

3.1a. What is this problem?
3.1b. What control measures may assist the herd?

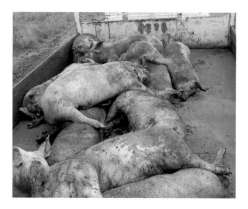

Fig. 3.1i. Numerous dead pigs with cyanosis of the ears and snout.

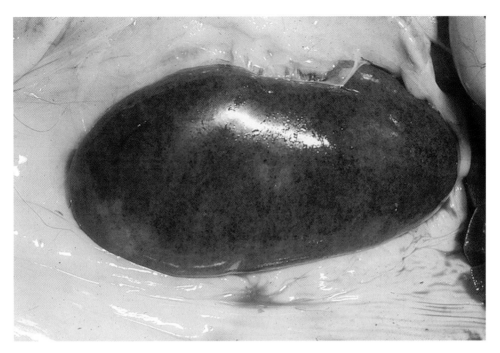

Fig. 3.1ii. Autopsy with haemorrhagic kidney and oedema fluid in abdomen.

3.1 Comments

3.1a. This is the current so-called Georgia form of African swine fever (ASF), which is caused by a highly contagious virus. The ASF virus and disease is specific to pigs and must be confirmed by testing of blood or tissues. ASF disease has been spreading and is uncontrolled across eastern areas of Europe. Throughout this time, the virus has remained highly virulent, that is, killing nearly all the pigs it contacts. The ASF virus is resistant to the environment and can survive in pig pens, pork products and dead pigs for some months. The spread of the disease has therefore been facilitated by infected pigs entering local markets and wandering pigs, and also by the feeding of food wastes (containing pork with ASF virus) to local pigs. This disease is now the major exotic threat to pig health and welfare across Asia and Europe.

3.1b. There are no treatments and no vaccines for ASF, therefore this fatal disease is of great concern to all pig farmers around the world. All people across the pig industry must study video and other training aids to correctly suspect and identify this major threat. ASF is highly contagious and is on the World Organisation for Animal Health (OIE) list A of international trade (this indicates that this is a notifiable disease with the potential for serious and rapid spread and there are restrictions on international trade of animals and animal products). In an outbreak, nearly all pigs are usually affected and they will provide a source of infection for other animals. Any suspicion of ASF should lead to the farmer calling the government authorities, who may stop all movement of people and animals on and off the farm. Samples of tissues and blood samples must be sent to designated laboratories in secure packaging for virus isolation and identification. All dead pigs must be processed for proper disposal so that the resistant virus is not transmitted from this source.

3.2 Case Study

The farmer operated an established nursery and finisher pig farm system, which received weaner pigs from local breeder farms, with modern lines of pig breeds. The breeder pigs and young piglets all received a complete vaccination programme. The grower pigs were raised in older-style buildings, each housing several hundred pigs in various pens. The pig feeds were prepared in a wet-meal form with cereals, soybean and some by-products. The growing pigs were usually fed meals twice a day, at various times, depending on staff schedules. The pigs were highly active when each meal was delivered into the older-style feeder boxes inside the pens (Fig. 3.2i). The farmer noticed that for several months, many batches of growing pigs had higher mortality levels. Close inspection indicated that 2–5% of the 10–20-week-old pigs in the grower and finisher period had died, usually at the rate of a few pigs per week. The farm workers reported that these pigs usually died suddenly and that they only occasionally noticed a pig just prior to its death. These dying pigs were depressed and inactive, with a hunched abdomen. At autopsy of the affected pigs, the pigs were pale with a greatly swollen abdomen. When the abdomen was carefully opened up, many loops of intestine were seen to be greatly enlarged and swollen with smelly gas and bloody fluid contents (Fig. 3.2ii). These loops of intestine were in various bright colours ranging from purple to green. When the veterinarian reached under these loops, to the base of the intestine at the spine, the intestine loops were found to be twisted into a tight knot.

Key Features

- Numerous sporadic and sudden deaths in active grower pigs.
- Twisted and swollen intestinal loops in abdomen.

3.2a. What is this problem?
3.2b. What control measures may assist the herd?

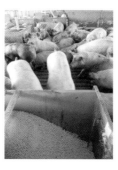

Fig. 3.2i. Active pigs at feeders in pens.

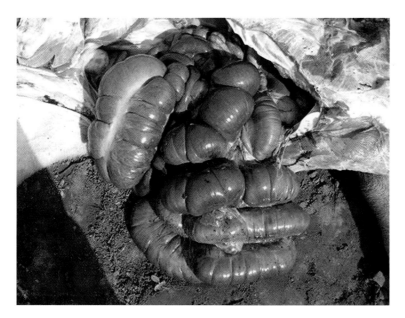

Fig. 3.2ii. Twisted and swollen intestinal loops in abdomen.

3.2 Comments

3.2a. This condition is twisting or torsion of the intestines in growing pigs. The small intestinal tract of the pig is quite long, usually measuring 15 times the length of the body. It is connected to the pig's body by a connective tissue mesh known as the mesentery, which hangs loose from the roof of the abdomen in a standing pig. In active grower pigs, this means that twists and torsions of the small intestine can occur commonly, which can quickly result in an extreme intestinal accident, stopping the blood supply and quickly killing the pig. It is therefore very important that any investigation of the cause of sudden death in a pig includes a palpation of the root of the mesentery, to check for intestinal torsion. It is a common condition in modern pig farms around the world. It is often seen in active grower pigs where there is excessive activity, falling about and competitive jousting and overeating at the feeding areas. This behaviour problem is exacerbated if there are erratic feeding times and feeders that can accumulate feed in certain areas. The case study presents a typical situation, but the mortality problem can be greatly increased if pigs are fed dairy by-products that also ferment inside the pig intestines.

3.2b. The problem of sporadic mortality due to torsions can be difficult to resolve and control measures revolve around management of feeding practices for the active growing pigs, to prevent rapid overeating. The stocking rate needs to be suitable for the feeders. The time interval between feed schedules in grower pigs needs to be steady, including at periods such as staff vacations. The feeders need to be managed so that piles of feed do not accumulate. The feeders need to be positioned at a level so that pigs do not fall about them. Some lines of pigs appear to be more active and aggressive at feeding times.

3.3 Case Study

The farmer operated a large, established breeder, nursery and finisher pig farm system. There were many smaller pig farms in the region and some of the farm workers kept pigs in their backyard settings at home. The farmer also occasionally purchased sows and nursery pigs from these local farms. The farmer had experienced a range of disease problems, and therefore used a lot of pig treatments, but he was concerned about farm costs and did not use many commercial vaccines. The farmer noticed a rapid increase in mortality in the pigs in several finisher sheds, rising to 40% mortality over a period of 1–2 weeks (Fig. 3.3i). Close inspection indicated that the dead and dying pigs had a dark congestion and blackened colour to their ears and snouts, known as cyanosis. Many of these pigs were dull and listless. Pigs seemed to slowly wander around in an aimless manner – the pig has nowhere to go and is in no hurry to get there. The pigs tended to lie down and huddle in piles. Many pigs also had sticky dark discharges noticeable at their eyes. Some pigs appeared to have yellow diarrhoea and vomiting. At autopsy of the dead pigs, there were bloody haemorrhages noticed in many of the lymph nodes and inside the urinary bladder. The kidneys seemed pale, with many small bloody spots on the surface (Fig. 3.3ii). The spleen was nearly normal size but had some rough dark areas at the edges. Blood tests showed that the pigs had a low white blood cell count (leukopenia).

Key Features

- Outbreak of high mortality rates in groups of pigs.
- Conjunctivitis and haemorrhages in lymph nodes in affected pigs.

3.3a. What is this problem?
3.3b. What control measures may assist the herd?

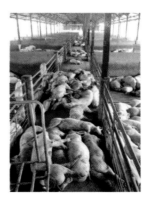

Fig. 3.3i. Numerous dead and dying pigs on the affected finisher sites.

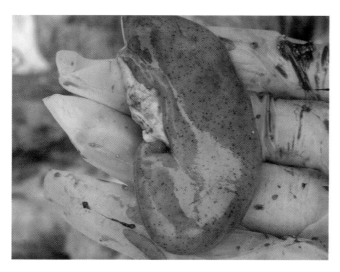

Fig. 3.3ii. Autopsy of dead pigs, with pale spotty kidneys.

3.3 Comments

3.3a. The high mortality and the autopsy signs are suggestive of CSF, which is caused by a pestivirus. CSF is also known as hog cholera in some countries. The case study illustrates the arrival of CSF on to a farm with low levels of immunity, where all the pigs are susceptible to a virulent strain of the virus and many deaths occur. In the pigs that survive and in later groups of infected pigs, CSF is often known as a 'great imitator' as the clinical signs in the sick pigs are often vague or inconclusive and may resemble other diseases. CSF can be confirmed by blood tests and virus tests such as PCR.

3.3b. Affected pigs do not respond well to antibiotics or other treatments. A vaccination programme must be implemented for farms that are positive for CSF. Commercial vaccines exist for CSF in many regions. A course of different CSF vaccines from international suppliers, such as the live attenuated C strain and the subunit E2 vaccines, should be implemented. Full protection against this disease in farms located in endemic and high-risk pig farming areas can be difficult, even with these vaccination programmes. This is due to the fact that the disease is very common and pigs may be exposed early in life, so the vaccine administration may actually occur at around the same time as the pigs are exposed to wild virus and while there is still some interference to protection from maternal antibodies. On many farms in this situation, it is therefore often necessary to develop multiple vaccine points around the time of weaning and during the early grower period.

The general effort required to keep diseases out, or manage their entry in a practical manner, is known as external biosecurity. The various factors that must be managed by farm owners in this effort to keep out CSF are: (i) consideration of the purchase of replacement pigs and semen; (ii) the control of staff and visitors; and (iii) the entry of pigs, vehicles, equipment and pork product on to farms. In this case study, it is possible that farm workers may have introduced the infection on to the larger farm from their backyard pigs, via boots, clothing or perhaps pork products. It is vital that all pork products are excluded from pig farm areas, including canteens. It is important not to allow farm workers or visitors to provide any outside food waste to farm pigs.

3.4 Case Study

The farmer operated an established nursery and finisher pig farm system. The farm received weaner pigs from local breeder farms with modern lines of pig breeds. The breeder pigs and young piglets all received a complete vaccination programme. The grower pigs were raised in groups of modern buildings, each housing several hundred pigs. The pig feeds were prepared in a high-density pelleted form by a large feed mill, with cereal, soybeans and vitamin and mineral additive components (Fig. 3.4i). The feed mill used a fine particle-size mesh to prepare the high-density pellets, to ensure that the feed pellets did not crumble apart during transport and storage. The growing pigs were usually fed meals twice a day. The farmer noticed that during the hot summer months many batches of growing pigs around 10–18 weeks old had several pigs with lethargy and there were some deaths in the groups. Close inspection indicated that some individual pigs were lethargic, coughing and with some dark bloody patches on their faeces. They also occasionally showed abdominal pain by kicking at their abdomen. The groups of pigs showed few other clear signs apart from these few sick pigs, but with an increased mortality in the group. At autopsy of these dead pigs, the pigs were pale and in good body condition. When the stomach was opened, it was found to contain a large amount of blood-clot material (Fig. 3.4ii). There was deep ulceration around the oesophageal opening to the stomach. This ulcer had a smooth, rolled and raised border. The floor of the ulcer had a rough, bile-stained appearance. The intestines of the pigs were normal, but some pigs had pneumonia in the lungs.

Key Features

- Pelleted pig-feed preparation and interruptions in feed intake.
- Pale pig with ulcerated oesophago-gastric area of stomach.

3.4a. What is this problem?
3.4b. What control measures may assist the herd?

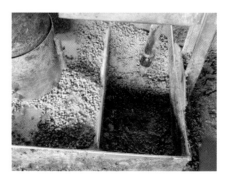

Fig. 3.4i. Pelleted pig feed preparation.

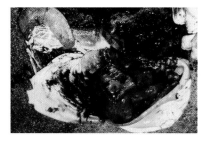

Fig. 3.4ii. Ulcerated oesophago-gastric area of the stomach with bloody contents.

3.4 Comments

3.4a. This is death due to ulceration of the pars oesophagea of the pig stomach, associated with a rapid rupture of local blood vessels in the ulcer and death due to anaemia and blood loss. Oesophageal gastric ulceration (OGU) is a common problem on many modern pig farms around the world. The pig has a monogastric stomach, but this organ has several distinctive features that predispose pigs to OGU. A rectangular-shaped zone in the stomach lining of the lesser curvature is known as the pars oesophagea. It surrounds the oesophageal opening and extends to the rear. The glands of the stomach that secrete acid and protein enzyme (pepsin) are located in the other areas of the stomach. OGU is not an infectious disease; it is an attack on the pars oesophagea by the acid normally found in the other parts of the stomach. This attack is caused by a combination of two factors. First, the diet consisting of fine particles of pelleted feed fills the stomach with suspensions of acid and feed. Secondly, these pigs have had an interruption to their normal daily feed intake, which makes the acid-feed suspension rise up to the pars oesophagea zone and attack it. In this case study, the interruption may have been due to the hot summer weather. Hot temperatures inside pig pens invariably makes the pigs reluctant to move around and eat properly. This interruption to feed intake can also occur for many other reasons, such as: (i) poor care of the feeders in pens; (ii) a health problem; (iii) overcrowding; (iv) the addition of some poorly palatable feed item; or (v) poor air quality due to ventilation problems. Pigs with OGU at low levels are often associated with some pneumonia and coughing.

3.4b. Pigs may be treated for OGU with the anti-stomach acid drug, ranitidine. This drug is available in various formulations, such as syrups, which may be given to pigs. It can be difficult to alter the background factors behind OGU cases, because pelleted feed is highly suitable for larger-scale operations and short cessations in feed intake can occur in groups of pigs, for many reasons on most farms. Feed mills and farmers prefer high-density pelleted feed with fine particles (such as a 400 μm mesh in the feed mill), because it does not crumble when handled and gives a high energy intake and growth rate to the pigs. The control of OGU on a broader basis requires attention to feed quality, consistency and particle size. A larger particle size and increased roughage may be added to the feed mix. It is also important to pay attention to the various factors that may cause pigs to cease feed intake, even on an intermittent basis. This may be addressed by: (i) better temperature control in hot weather; (ii) appropriate stocking density and feeder spaces; (iii) removal of any poorly palatable feed item; and (iv) control of ongoing disease problems.

3.5   Case Study

The farmer operated an established breeder, nursery and finisher farm system with several older-style buildings, some straw-bedding floor areas and some open, outdoor pens. Some finisher and breeder pigs were put in the outdoor pens for the early summer months. The farmer provided plenty of feed and water outlets for the pigs. The older buildings had populations of rodents and bird numbers in and around the areas for housing pigs. The farmer operated a minimal medication and vaccination programme for the pigs. The farmer noticed that several grower and finisher pigs over the period of the hot summer months had become sick and were in poor condition (Fig. 3.5i). Close inspection indicated that the affected sick pigs were of various ages, from 12 to 25 weeks old. The pigs moved about slowly in a stiff manner and were dull and depressed, but did not have signs of diarrhoea or coughing. Some of these sick pigs had become duller, had stopped moving around or eating and a few pigs had died. Many of the sick pigs developed several distinctive diamond-shaped circumscribed plaque-like lesions on the skin of their back, flanks and shoulders (Fig. 3.5ii). At autopsy of some of the pigs that died, as well as the skin lesions, there was some cyanosis over the ears and snout, with a few haemorrhages in the spleen, lymph nodes and kidneys.

Key Features

- Sick pigs of various ages.
- Diamond-shaped rhomboid lesions on the skin of the flank of sick pigs.

3.5a. What is this problem?
3.5b. What control measures may assist the herd?

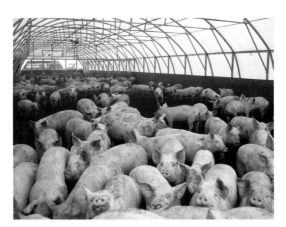

Fig. 3.5i. Sick finisher pigs with straw-bedding floor areas.

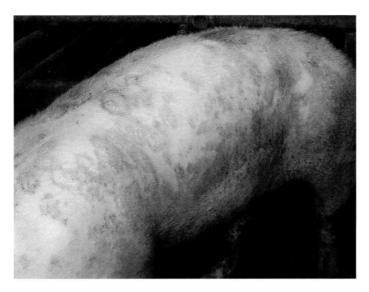

Fig. 3.5ii. Diamond-shaped lesions on the skin of the flank of sick pigs.

3.5 Comments

3.5a. This condition is the common form of erysipelas, a disease of pigs caused by the bacterium *Erysipelothrix* sp. The distinctive skin lesions are an unforgettable diagnostic feature of this disease in pigs. Erysipelas is a common disease on pig farms around the world. The clinical disease often occurs in low numbers among older production pigs on many farms, but with occasional outbreaks affecting many pigs among groups of nursery, grower or finisher or breeder pigs on some farms. The main source of infections and outbreaks of erysipelas for pigs is usually some form of steady build-up of the bacterium in the environment of the pigs, such as the soil of outdoor pens, dirty buildings or bedding materials, or via farm pigs, rodents or birds that are carrying and spreading a heavy load of the bacterium to some groups of pigs around a farm building.

3.5b. Pigs that are suffering the more severe clinical forms of the disease can be rapidly and effectively treated with penicillin antibiotic products. As with all treatment programmes, best results are obtained if the treatment is given at an early stage of the problem. It is also often necessary to provide penicillin medication to the entire group of pigs via drinking water or in the feed.

A range of commercial vaccines exist for erysipelas and are required as part of a complete vaccination programme for all breeder pigs (i.e. gilts, sows and boars). Vaccination is best given in two doses to the sows and gilts in late pregnancy, 3 weeks prior to farrowing. Booster vaccines are often required for breeder pigs every 6 months. Many farms with indoor pigs do not need to vaccinate the production piglets or grower pigs, unless there have been outbreaks in an established farm setting.

Attention to farm hygiene and pest control are also important to reduce the environmental load of the bacterium. Removal of straw bedding and outdoor pen systems and replacement with indoor, slatted-concrete floor systems will greatly reduce erysipelas problems for the pigs.

3.6   Case Study

The farmer operated a medium-sized farm system with breeder, nursery and finisher units on a single large farm site. There were many other similar farms in the region. The farmer had purchased many gilts and developed various new lines of modern pig breeds and housed the nursery and finisher pigs in various new and older buildings. The performance of the breeder farm was poor, with a number of abortions noted and low numbers of pigs born alive. The farmer also noticed that over a period of 1 year the mortality rate among many of the groups of nursery, grower and finisher pigs was high (Fig. 3.6i). Close inspection indicated that the mortality started to increase in most of the groups at somewhere between 10–18 weeks old. Some of these pigs were noticed to have a mild cough, but this was variable between pigs. Occasionally, several pigs would die in a group in a 1 week period. Generally, the grower and finisher pigs seemed to be depressed with poor appetite and in poor body condition and were slow at getting to slaughter weight. At autopsy of the dead pigs, a wide range of problems was noted. In some pigs, there was a diffuse firmness and a mottled, tan colour to all the lobes of the lungs, including the front and rear lobes (Fig. 3.6ii). In some pigs, there were also areas of fibrin and pleurisy over some areas of the front lobes. In some other pigs, there was inflammation of the lining of the abdomen, known as peritonitis. In some other pigs, there was a necrotic enteritis. The problems continued to persist for many months and did not respond to antibiotic and other medications.

Key Features

- High mortality rates in nursery, grower and finisher areas.
- Range of problems found in dead pigs at autopsy.

3.6a. What is this problem?
3.6b. What control measures may assist the herd?

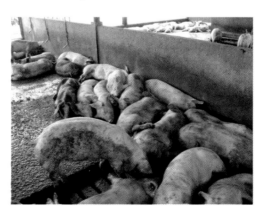

Fig. 3.6i. Groups of dull and dying grower pigs.

3.6   Comments

3.6a. This is a general mortality disease situation in farms that have ongoing infections and problems with the PRRS virus. Since its emergence in the 1980s, this virus has become the number one health problem facing pigs around the world. The PRRS virus is a common infection in pigs and has many strains. The PRRS virus is carried in the wind and is easily inhaled by pigs from the excretions of infected pigs. It is infectious even in small doses and from all secretions of pigs (saliva, faeces, aerosol, semen).

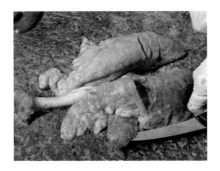

Fig. 3.6ii. Lung lesions in affected pigs.

There is commonly cross-transmission between different age groups, such as from breeder pigs to nursery pigs. In nursery and grower pigs, it can cause a direct interstitial pneumonia; this is a type of pneumonia that attacks the blood vessels and linings of the airways in the lungs. Another part of the basis of the strong hold that PRRS has over pigs is its ability to attack and harm the macrophages in the lungs. These cells are the ones that normally roam around the surfaces of the lungs grabbing and killing viruses and bacteria that enter the lungs, when the pig takes in inspired air. So an outbreak of PRRS infections in a group of pigs can have many consequences for the respiratory system. This will include diffuse pneumonia and also common secondary infections caused by other viruses and bacteria. So a farm with PRRS infections will commonly have a range of diseases and raised mortality rates.

3.6b. The various secondary infections in PRDC, such as swine influenza, need to be considered for vaccination and medication programmes. The underlying PRRS virus has proved difficult to control, particularly in areas where there are many pig farms in nearby areas. Because there are many strains, and new strains are continually evolving, having a recent outbreak of PRRS does not provide any immunity to the next PRRS virus entry and disease outbreak. It is therefore a common and ongoing problem.

It has proved possible to eradicate PRRS infections from breeding farms, by operating a completely closed herd and waiting for immunity to develop in the sows. After some months, these immune sows can then be inseminated with PRRS-negative semen and produce PRRS-negative litters of piglets. These piglets may be raised to become PRRS negative nursery and grower pigs, if they are also kept fully isolated from other pigs. For a farm system to use this process requires good isolation of the farm sites and prevention of new infections in the future. It is therefore difficult to follow this programme in an area with many other pig farms nearby.

The control of PRRS therefore often relies on vaccines. Various PRRS vaccines are available. The modified live PRRS vaccines have been useful at providing some protection to pigs, which may be exposed to PRRS virus strains similar to the ones present in the vaccine. It is often important to establish what strain of PRRS virus is on the pig farm. This usually requires the use of PCR tests. For control of respiratory disease due to PRRS, the vaccine may be applied to piglets at 3 weeks old. However, current vaccines do not prevent infections with all PRRS strains and disease can still occur in vaccinated pigs.

3.7 Case Study

The farmer operated an established medium-sized breeder farm, which had a mixture of newer and older buildings. The farmer used a complete vaccination programme for the breeding pigs. The farm received large batches of feed deliveries from a local feed mill. Many of the breeder pigs were housed in individual stalls and the farm staff filled the feed troughs of the sows once a day, by hand. The farm had modern lines of pig breeds and the farrowing rate and numbers of pigs born alive were at the target levels. The farmer noticed that the mortality levels of the breeder sows and gilts and some of the boars rose noticeably, following periods when the type of feed was changed to a low-fibre formulation. Close inspection indicated that these dead breeders had died suddenly, in good body condition. The dead pig was a normal colour, but the abdomen of the pig was hugely distended like an enormous balloon (Fig. 3.7i). When the abdomen was carefully opened, the distension was found to be due to massive dilation of the stomach of the pig, filled largely with smelly gas, but also with partly digested feed and watery fluid contents (Fig. 3.7ii). In some pigs, the stomach appeared to have partly twisted, allowing the spleen to be readily viewed lying on top of the stomach. The lungs of the pigs were very dark and filled with blood.

Key Features

- Deaths in breeder pigs with enlarged abdomen.
- Dilated gas-filled stomach in dead breeder pig.

3.7a. What is this problem?
3.7b. What control measures may assist the herd?

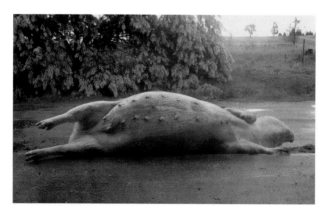

Fig. 3.7i. Dead breeder pig with enlarged abdomen.

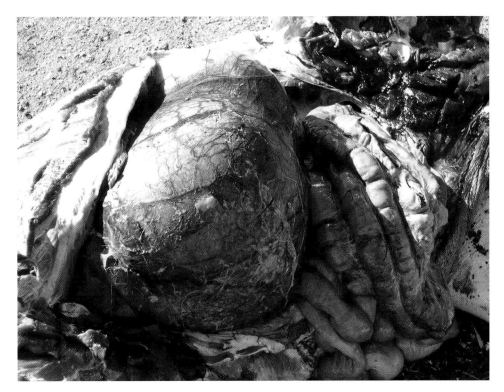

Fig. 3.7ii. Dilated gas-filled stomach in dead breeder pig.

3.7 Comments

3.7a. This condition is gastric dilation (i.e. massive dilation of the stomach of pigs). The huge dilation and firm enlargement of the stomach, mainly with gas, leads to pressure on the blood vessels, lungs and heart of the pig, causing failure of blood flow and death. It usually affects breeder pigs and is a common problem on many modern breeder farms around the world. It appears to be more common when pigs are shifted on to low-fibre diets, particularly when the breeder pigs are fed once a day and do not gain much exercise, such as when they are in individual stalls or in lactation. In this situation, some of the sows will rapidly eat a large amount of soft food, mixed with air, that becomes fermented in the stomach, producing large amounts of gas. This excessive gas cannot be released, resulting in the massive stomach dilation. In most other feeding situations, food is not fermented in the stomach and any ingested gas may be regurgitated.

3.7b. There is no medical or other simple treatment for pigs suffering gastric dilation. The pigs at risk of gastric dilation should be given access to cereal straw, bran or other high-fibre material, which usually will act to reduce the risk of fermentation of the normal diet. It is also recommended to feed breeder pigs at least twice a day, to reduce the amount of soft feed entering the stomach at any one time.

3.8 Case Study

The farmer operated an established nursery, grower and finisher pig farm system, with a mixture of new and older buildings. The farm received weaner pigs in batches arriving on trucks from local breeder farms. The nursery-stage pigs received a complete medication and vaccination programme. The farmer had increased the numbers of weaner pigs arriving, with an increase in pig stocking rates in the pens in many of the buildings. During an extended period of autumn weather patterns, the farmer noticed an outbreak of deaths among groups of finisher pigs, mainly in the older buildings. Close inspection indicated that 20–40% of the 14–18-week-old finisher pigs in these crowded pens had rapidly become sick and died over a few days. The ventilation in these older buildings was poor and the room thermometers indicated wide fluctuations in temperatures, with hot days and cold nights. It was noticed that prior to death the affected finisher pigs were dull, sitting or lying on the ground, often with a foamy, bloody discharge from their mouth and nose (Fig. 3.8i). These pigs seemed to have difficulty breathing and some were coughing. At autopsy of the dead pigs, the farmer and veterinarian noticed some dark black, haemorrhagic patches scattered in both the front and the rear lobes of the lungs (Fig. 3.8ii). There was some discoloration over these patches, with a dark metallic sheen forming over the lungs and pleurisy over these areas.

Key Features

- Rapid increase in mortality in finisher pigs.
- Dark haemorrhagic patches in lung lobes.

3.8a. What is this problem?
3.8b. What control measures may assist the herd?

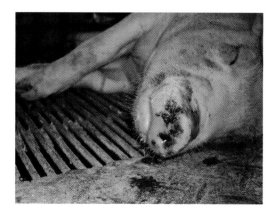

Fig. 3.8i. Numerous dead and dying pigs with foamy bloody nasal discharges.

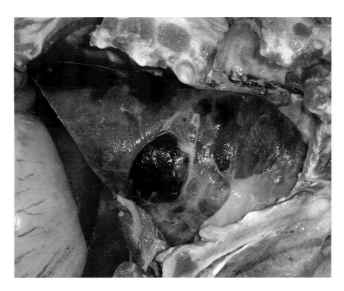

Fig. 3.8ii. Dark patches in the rear lobes of the lungs.

3.8 Comments

3.8a. This is the more acute form of pleuropneumonia caused by the bacterium *Actinobacillus pleuropneumoniae* (APP). Disease caused by APP is serious and common in pig farms around the world. The bacterium is present in most herds and has many toxins, which can have a strong debilitating effect on pig lungs. There are at least 15 known variants or serotypes of this APP bacterium. Many pig farms around the world are often infected with one of these serotypes, which are carried by sows in the breeder herd and transmitted to their piglet progeny. Some of these pigs will become fully infected after weaning and spread the disease quickly among the group. The outbreaks of severe acute APP in groups of finisher pigs will occur commonly when pigs are infected with a damaging serotype, and the pigs are overcrowded, in older buildings with poor ventilation. The APP disease is very harmful to farm economics, because of the loss of finisher pigs, which have had considerable investment already placed in them, prior to sale. Outbreaks can occur just prior to sending late finisher pigs to slaughter. Some of the 15 APP serotypes are milder and may only cause a less fatal pneumonia disease, with coughing as the main feature.

3.8b. Treatment of affected pigs needs to be rapidly commenced via the use of injectable antibiotics, such as florfenicol, delivered to sick and coughing pigs. APP remains a common disease around the world affecting groups of finisher pigs. The APP bacterium is not easily removed from all pigs in groups by medications or vaccinations. APP has therefore not been reduced by the development of modern pig farm systems with purpose-built farm buildings, all-in, all-out batches and multiple site operations. The current commercial APP vaccines have not proved particularly useful at fully controlling the disease in all farm situations. Autogenous vaccines may be prepared from specific APP variants present on each farm, but this is a tedious procedure. Attention to improved ventilation of farm buildings and strategic use of in-feed antibiotics such as penicillin or tiamulin can help reduce the impact of the disease in most groups of pigs on an infected farm.

3.9 Case Study

The farmer operated an established medium-sized breeder, nursery and finisher farm system. The farm was located in a region with many other pig farms nearby. The progeny were raised through the nursery phase in weekly batches to the grower and finisher stages. The farmer conducted a complete medication and vaccination programme for the breeder pigs and production pigs. The farrowing rates and numbers born alive were at the target levels. The farmer noticed an increase in moderate numbers of sick and dying pigs in the grower and finisher stage, with pigs affected at 11–15 weeks old, over a period of several weeks. Close inspection indicated that these sick pigs had poor appetite and were dull and depressed, with loss of growth and condition. Some of these dull and depressed pigs had some purple–blue discoloration of their ears, snout and legs (cyanosis) (Fig. 3.9i). These sick pigs often proceeded to become moribund and died. Deaths among the batches of 11–15-week-old age group increased by 5–15%. Some of the older pigs also showed signs of coughing and weight loss. The problem seemed to ease once the pigs reached 18–20 weeks old and the mortality in this older group was at a normal rate. At autopsy of the dead pigs, the farmer and veterinarian noticed that there was an empty stomach, noticeable enlargement of the liver and spleen and haemorrhages in the lymph nodes (Fig. 3.9ii). The most prominent sign was a blue–grey discoloration of the lungs, with a firm rubbery texture throughout and a thick mucoid exudate in the airways.

Key Features

- Moderate levels of cyanosis and deaths of grower and finisher pigs.
- Lung lesions and enlarged liver/spleen at autopsy.

3.9a. What is this problem?
3.9b. What control measures may assist the herd?

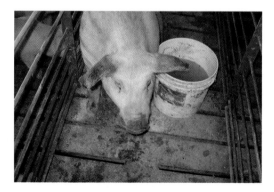

Fig. 3.9i. Cyanosis in some sick affected pigs.

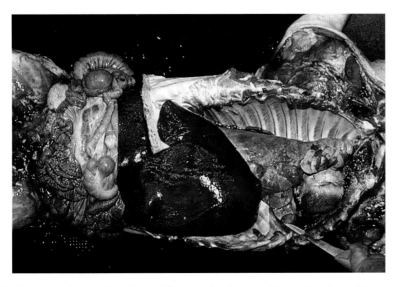

Fig. 3.9ii. Autopsy of pig with enlarged liver and spleen and firm discoloured lungs.

3.9 Comments

3.9a. This is a typical case history for an outbreak of infection by the bacterium *Salmonella cholerae-suis*. This particular strain of Salmonella is adapted to pigs, and is one member of a group of Salmonella known as Group C. Because this strain is adapted to pigs, it forms a general infection throughout the body of infected pigs, including the lungs, liver and spleen. This leads to the clinical signs of sick pigs, with some deaths. It is therefore important to culture the Salmonella from cases of sick pigs by sending samples from the dead pigs to a bacteriology laboratory. Many pig farms are negative for *S. cholerae-suis* so the disease is not a common problem in modern pig farms. There have only been occasional outbreaks in pig farms reported around the world in the past decades.

There are many other strains of the Salmonella bacteria and most of them cause infections in the intestines of animals, including pigs. In some situations, these Salmonella infections in the intestines can cause diarrhoea problems for infected pigs. Salmonella infections of all strains in pigs are more likely to be significant on pig farms that are also positive for PCV-2 or CSF.

3.9b. Grower pigs that are infected with *S. cholerae-suis* may be treated with antibiotic medications in the feed or water. It is appropriate to medicate the pigs for at least 2 weeks. Salmonella infections are difficult to control, and the infection can persist on pig farms for long periods. Many Salmonella are resistant to some antibiotics, so the use of many different antibiotics on farms does not always reduce the infection in the herd. Salmonella vaccines have not been particularly useful for control of the infection or disease on farms. Control measures for PCV-2 and CSF should also be checked and improved by vaccination. The most useful measure for control of Salmonella is therefore improvement of farm hygiene, with cleaning of manure pits, walkways and control of rodents and birds on the farm site.

3.10 Case Study

The farmer operated a medium-sized breeder farm, with sows and boars from modern lines of pig breeds. The farrowing rate and numbers of piglets born alive were at the target levels. Pigs were housed in mating, gestation and lactation pens, in modern well-constructed buildings. The farmer noticed that over the past year, an occasional adult sow or adult boar would appear sick and suffer a loss of body condition. The individual pigs did not respond to antibiotics or other medication and died after being sick for some days (Fig. 3.10i). Other pigs in the same pens and rooms appeared normal. At autopsy of these individual dead pigs, there were spectacular lesions of an enlarged liver, which had numerous large yellow cheese-like caseous nodules present (Fig. 3.10ii). These prominent nodules were also visible in the lymph nodes and all the lobes of the lungs.

Key Features

- Occasional death of adult pig.
- Large nodules in the lungs and liver.

3.10a. What is this problem?
3.10b. What control measures may assist the herd?

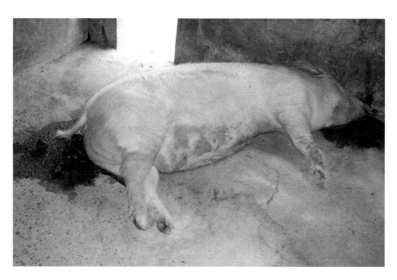

Fig. 3.10i. Occasional dead adult pig.

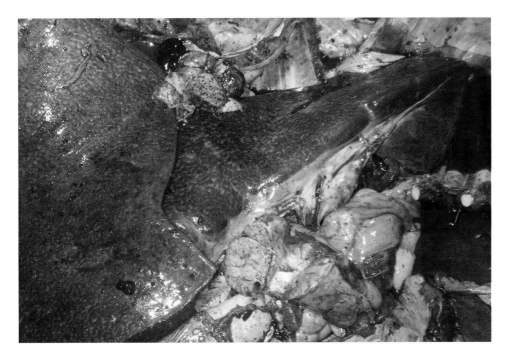

Fig. 3.10ii. Large nodules in the lymph nodes and liver of a dead pig.

3.10   Comments

3.10a. This is a case of the most common form of cancer or neoplasia in the pig, known as a lymphoma. This is a cancerous growth of the lymphoid cells of the pig, which form the large growths or nodules in the liver and lungs. Cancer in pigs is not infectious and usually is seen as an occasional death of an adult sow or boar, as in this case study. It does not cause outbreaks of disease or deaths. The formation of cheese-like nodules in the liver or lungs of pigs can be confused with cases of tuberculosis caused by Mycobacteria, so it is important that specimens are sampled and examined by a pathology laboratory.

3.10b. Lymphoma cancer in pigs cannot be treated or prevented by current technology. It is important for an autopsy of pigs to be carried out by veterinarians in collaboration with the farmer, so that cases of individual diseases, such as cancer, which do not threaten the herd, can be contrasted with many other diseases, which may be infectious and threaten other pigs.

3.11   Case Study

The farmer operated an established farm system with breeder, nursery and finisher units, with various older-style buildings. The pens in some buildings had a mixture of older-style wooden and concrete slats and floors. The breeder pigs and young piglets all received a complete vaccination programme. The breeding farm had a variety of modern pig breeds. However, the farmer had few staff and hygiene levels in the piglet processing areas (where teeth clipping, tail docking and injections took place) were not optimal. The weaned pigs from the breeder farm areas were moved to a nursery production pig area at 3–4 weeks old. The farmer noticed an ongoing problem of occasional deaths among the various groups of pigs (Fig. 3.11i). Close inspection indicated that affected individual pigs were in a wide age range of 8–16 weeks old; they were seen to be dull and sick for a few days, then became weak, with some purple–blue discoloration of the body, then died. The other pigs in the pens were normal. At autopsy of these dead pigs, the farmer and veterinarian noticed lesions consistent with death due to heart failure, with an enlarged, blood-filled liver and lots of pale fluid in the lungs. When the cavity of the heart was opened, the main heart valves were greatly thickened, reddened and distorted with dull, cauliflower-shaped, crumbly masses (Fig. 3.11ii).

Key Features

- Occasional deaths in production pigs.
- Autopsy shows dull, cauliflower-shaped masses on the heart valves.

3.11a. What is this problem?
3.11b. What control measures may assist the herd?

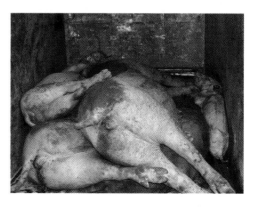

Fig. 3.11i. Deaths of occasional nursery and grower and finisher pigs.

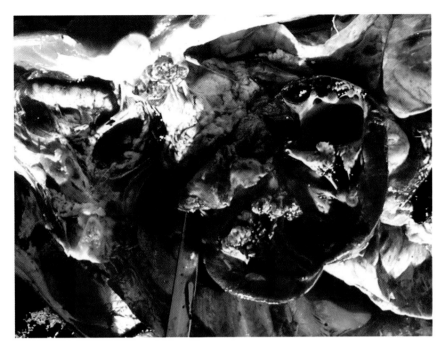

Fig. 3.11ii. Dull, cauliflower-shaped masses on the valves of the heart.

3.11 Comments

3.11a. This condition is known as valvular endocarditis. It occurs, usually at a low level, on most pig farms around the world. The affected pigs usually do not show any specific signs before death and the diagnosis is made at autopsy. The condition occurs when a bacterial infection in the bloodstream of the pig becomes settled on to the valves of the heart. This bacterial growth becomes large and inflamed and eventually leads to failure of the function of the heart valves, leading to heart failure with poor blood flow through the major organs, such as the liver and lungs. The specific bacteria that settle down on the heart valves and cause this disease may not always be clearly identified. In some cases, the bacteria may be identified as being *Streptococcus* sp. or the agent of erysipelas. The original source of these bacteria into the bloodstream is often from poor management practices. These poor management practices may allow small wounds of young piglets to become contaminated. This can be from dirty equipment used to clip teeth or tails, dirty injection needles or from small injuries to the pigs' feet from older floor types.

3.11b. There are no reliable medication or vaccination programmes that will specifically address valvular endocarditis. The problem is often at a low level on most farms, which does not justify major interventions. The hygiene of all processing equipment and staff training to maintain all hygiene measures must be addressed. It is important that cleansing of teeth clippers occurs between pigs and two separate clean and sharp instruments are used to clip teeth and dock tails – *never* the same one for these two procedures. Floors, doors and walls of pig pens need to be free of any sections likely to injure the young pigs.

3.12   Case Study

The farmer operated a large farm with several sheds and open pasture lands. The pig farm was located in an agricultural region with many outdoor livestock farms nearby, including long-established cattle and sheep farms. The pig farmer had purchased some of these lands and developed some outdoor spaces for groups of breeding and finisher pigs from his sheds. The farmer provided plenty of feed and water outlets for these roaming outdoor pigs. The weather had some dry spells while the pigs were in these outdoor spaces. The farmer noticed that over a period of several weeks, some of the finisher pigs in the dry pastures were listless and dull, with some swelling around their neck. Close inspection indicated that the affected pigs were older growers and finisher pigs. These pigs were dull, not eating, with a firm, hot and painful swelling across their throat, neck and lower face. This swelling caused the pigs to have trouble breathing, taking noisy breaths and not eating properly. Many of these pigs had died a few days after these signs had been noticed (Fig. 3.12i). Some other pigs had dark bloody diarrhoea. At autopsy, the pigs with the swollen throat (Fig. 3.12ii) had firm gelatinous oedema fluid in the neck, with extensive infiltration of neck and jaw tissues with clear, bloody wine-like fluid and gelatinous material. The local lymph nodes were greatly enlarged and oedematous. The internal organs including the liver and spleen appeared relatively normal.

Key Features

- Pigs with swollen throat and difficulty breathing.
- Autopsy of dead pigs shows enlarged gelatinous swelling in neck and lymph nodes.

3.12a. What is this problem?
3.12b. What control measures may assist the herd?

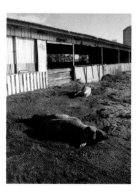

Fig. 3.12i. Dead pigs in the outdoor area.

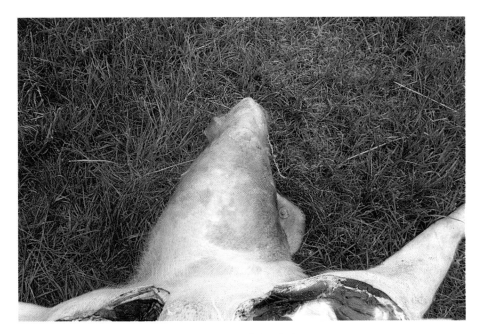

Fig. 3.12ii. Large swelling in throat and neck of dead pig.

3.12 Comments

3.12a. This condition is the typical presentation in pigs of the ancient animal disease known as anthrax, caused by the large bacterium *Bacillus anthracis*. This bacterium occurs in the soil only in defined endemic regions, so it can enter the bloodstream of outdoor pigs that consume this soil. The bacterium then often settles in the lymph nodes around the pig's jaw. It is not common for pigs to be raised on pasture in anthrax-positive areas, so the disease is not common in pigs. However, when it is does occur, it is usually a major dramatic episode for the farm, because of the strong ability of anthrax to cause public fear in humans.

Infection in humans occurs when the dead pigs in this situation are subject to autopsy or dissection by unskilled workers who transfer blood from the affected pig into their own bloodstream, via knife cuts. While serious outbreaks and incidents of anthrax infections in humans from this source occur globally, they are sporadic. It is important to confirm any suspicious deaths as being due to anthrax. This is done by staining and examination of dry smears of the lymph node and dark fluids in the neck. This diagnosis is not always simple, as the bacillus is often not present in the blood of infected pigs and the lymph node smears can be difficult to interpret in pigs, because the bacillus capsule is thin, and many other similar bacteria such as Clostridia may be present. Pigs that have received antibiotics will have few bacteria in the smears. It is therefore important to confirm anthrax in pigs by culture of the lymph nodes in a bacteriology laboratory.

3.12b. It is not appropriate to treat the pigs with antibiotics, as this will prolong the outbreak of this major public health disease. It is often difficult to easily dispose of the affected farm pigs in a practical manner. In general, they should be destroyed on site by incineration.

PART 4
Nervous Signs in Pigs

4.1 Case Study

The farmer operated a large farm system with breeder farms linked to various production pig nursery and finisher units. The breeder pigs and young piglets all received a complete vaccination programme. The weaned pigs moved to nursery production pig sites at 3–4 weeks old. The farm system received feed for its production pigs from a large feed-mill operation in various phases – starter, grower and finisher feeds. This feed mill decided to reduce the in-feed doses of antibiotics and zinc oxide added to the post-weaning starter diets. Soon after this, the managers of the nursery sites noticed some nervous signs among many of the recently weaned pigs. There was also a moderate increase in the mortality levels for the nursery period. Close examination indicated numerous weaner pigs displayed a range of nervous signs and depression. These clinical signs usually started 7–14 days after weaning from the sow, and seemed to affect particularly the larger and better-growing pigs. The nervous signs included uncoordinated ataxia (stumbling about), recumbency (lying down) and convulsions. Besides the nervous signs, many of the sick pigs had marked soft tissue swelling (oedema) of the upper and lower eyelids (Fig. 4.1i). Some affected pigs also had an amazing change in their normal vocalization sounds, from the usual strong squealing sound, into a high-pitch squeaky voice. At autopsy of some affected pigs, the soft gelatinous oedema was evident in the eyelids, but also in the area of the colon (Fig. 4.1ii), the wall of the stomach and the larynx.

Key Features

- Specific age range affected is 7–14 days after weaning.
- Wide range of nervous signs, including change in vocalization.
- Oedema of eyelids, stomach wall and colon.

4.1a. What is this problem?
4.1b. What control measures may assist the herd?

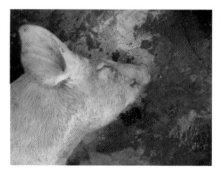

Fig. 4.1i. A 5-week-old weaner pig with recumbency and eyelid oedema.

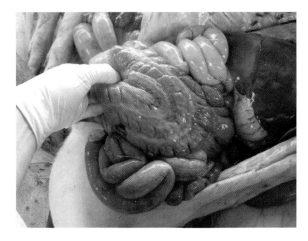

Fig. 4.1ii. Autopsy of affected nursery pig, with oedema of the colon.

4.1 Comments

4.1a. This is oedema disease of pigs, which is caused by strains of enterotoxigenic *Escherichia coli* (ETEC) bacteria that contain a specific vero-toxin (shiga-like toxin). These bacteria are located in the nursery-farm environment and are ingested by the piglet soon after weaning. The bacteria then attach to the small intestine and their toxins cause blood-vessel disturbances in the brain and other locations in the pig. The *E. coli* vaccines used in breeder pigs are aimed to provide immunity against ETEC in neonatal piglets and do not protect against ETEC infections in post-weaned pigs (i.e. once the pigs stop consuming milk and maternal antibodies). It is important to note that the infection with the toxigenic *E. coli* is inside the intestine (not in the brain) so the intestines of the pigs must be sampled to culture the correct strain of *E. coli*. Culture of intestine samples in a bacteriology laboratory will show heavy pure growth of the ETEC.

4.1b. Treatment of these piglets can be assisted with the antibiotic colistin, which is often regarded as the drug of choice, with no clear indication yet of resistance. Zinc oxide should be replaced back into the post-wean starter diets at pharmaceutical levels. *E. coli* and ETEC strains are a common background organism that is considered to be 'embedded' in most pig farms, presumably in materials in the pens, walkways and slurry. This embedded nature explains its constant nature of occurrence and outbreaks when appropriate control measures are not taken. The nursery areas that are old and dirty will be a reservoir of infection, if they are not cleaned properly. Cleaning of nursery areas must include the initial use of detergents, prior to use of washing and disinfectants. The amount of faeces material (slurry) underneath weaner pens needs to be managed properly.

The occurrence of clinical ETEC infections in post-weaned pigs has dropped away to a very low level since the 1980s with the introduction of in-feed zinc oxide at sufficient pharmaceutical levels (1500–3000 ppm) in early starter diets. Zinc oxide has a specific antibacterial action, damaging and distorting bacterial membranes with leakage of bacterial contents. In this case study, however, the reduction of zinc oxide usage away from appropriate pharmaceutical levels led quickly to outbreaks of clinical ETEC infections.

4.2   Case Study

The farmer operated an established medium-sized farm system with breeder, nursery and finisher units. The breeder pigs and young piglets all received a complete vaccination programme. The farm site had a variety of older buildings, with fixtures and pens in various stages of maintenance and repair. The pigs were given a mixed diet of commercial feeds and dairy by-products prepared on the farm. During a period of very cold weather, the farmer noticed that all the nursery-grower-age pigs in two adjacent pens were suddenly showing severe nervous signs. Close inspection indicated that many pigs were very agitated, jumping and bouncing around (Fig. 4.2i). Some pigs were gathered around their water drinkers (Fig. 4.2ii), other pigs wandered about aimlessly, and some appeared to press their head into walls. Several pigs were seen to walk backwards, and fall over backwards. Some more severely affected pigs were dull and had periods of convulsions. Several deaths had occurred in the first few hours of the incident. The walls and floors of the pens appeared very dry and no water was available when the drinkers in these pens were assessed.

Key Features

- Blockage to normal water supply with dry pens.
- Pigs with severe nervous signs, including backward-moving pigs.

4.2a. What is this problem?
4.2b. What control measures may assist the herd?

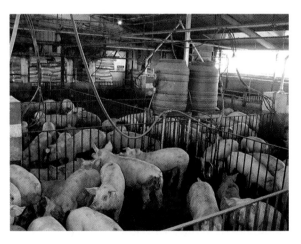

Fig. 4.2i. Agitated group of weaner-grower pigs with blocked water supply.

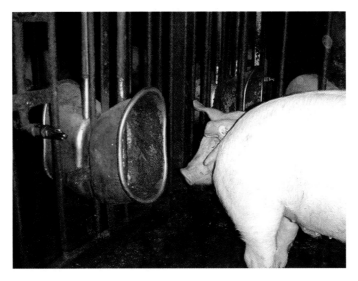

Fig. 4.2ii. Pigs gathered around empty water drinkers.

4.2   Comments

4.2a. This is a failure of the water supply to a group of pigs, leading to swelling of the brain and severe nervous signs. It remains a reasonably common incident on pig farms around the world. Pigs drink a lot of water and merely 24 h without a water supply will lead to deaths. Water-deprivation incidents commonly relate to an identifiable occurrence on the farm, such as: (i) frozen water pipes in a cold winter period; (ii) the blockage or failure of a header tank supplying water; or (iii) broken pipes within a building. The blockages of water tanks or pipes can occur due to dead rodents, straw materials or pipe deposits. Incidents can also occur due to staff negligence in operating the water supply, such as when water medications are introduced. The development of the nervous signs involves the build-up of salt in the brain, with water then entering the brain to cause the brain swelling inside the head. The problem is therefore often worse on high-salt diets, such as those with by-products. Most incidents of water deprivation in pigs, involve periods of more than 24 h without water supply.

4.2b. The treatment of pigs that have suffered water deprivation is very difficult. Quick restoration of water and rapid drinking can make the problem worse. Therefore affected pigs must have their water intake slowly restored in a limited way, with only small amounts of water given over the first day of treatment. Many pigs affected by water deprivation do not recover well, even when water is slowly resupplied.

The normal requirement for clean, accessible water by pigs is 10 l/100 kg bodyweight of growing pigs. Incidents of water deprivation will be prevented if water supplies are regularly checked and maintained properly. Pipes and water tanks need to be cleaned and maintained free of blockages. Pig farms should carry a spare tank of water for emergency pig supply if necessary. Pigs will require more water supply, when fed by-products and in hot weather.

4.3   Case Study

The farmer operated an established farm system with breeder, nursery and finisher units. The breeder pigs and young piglets all received a complete vaccination programme. The breeding farm had a successful programme of modern genetics, with different farm sites having a variety of modern pig breeds. The weaned pigs from the different breeder farm areas were moved to a nursery production pig area at 3–4 weeks old. The farmer noticed nervous signs in the weaner-stage pigs. A similar problem had been noted around 6 months previously. Close inspection indicated that affected pigs were 5–10 weeks old; they were seen to be dull and separate from the group, then collapse on to their side. These recumbent pigs then commenced intermittent but prolonged paddling of their front legs, with their head and back arched backwards (Fig. 4.3i). These paddling leg convulsions were seen in many affected pigs, and were sometimes stimulated by noise or handling. These pigs often did not recover and died. There was a noticeable increase in mortality of nursery-stage pigs, compared with the previous 3 months. Some affected sick pigs appeared to respond well to penicillin antibiotics. At autopsy of some affected pigs, the head of the pigs were carefully opened and some of the linings around the base of the brain stem appeared dull and cloudy, but no other changes were noted (Fig. 4.3ii).

Key Features

- Nursery-age pigs with nervous signs.
- Many affected pigs with paddling convulsions.

4.3a. What is this problem?
4.3b. What control measures may assist the herd?

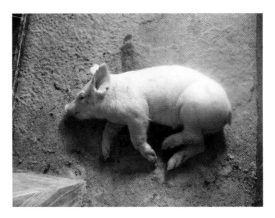

Fig. 4.3i. Weaner pig with paddling leg motions.

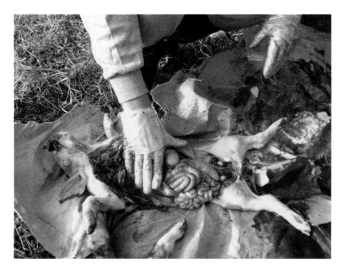

Fig. 4.3ii. Autopsy of affected nursery pig.

4.3 Comments

4.3a. This is inflammation of the linings of the brain or meningitis caused by the bacterium *Streptococcus suis*, which is a common bacterial infection in pigs. This bacterium lives in the environment of pig farms in dust and faeces in sheds and in carrier pigs. The clinical disease is common on many farms around the world, typically in a proportion of pigs some weeks after weaning. The problem tends to occur in sporadic outbreaks and can reappear after some change in management or medication programmes. The bacterium enters the bloodstream of some pigs and often settles in the brain, causing nervous convulsions and deaths. The *S. suis* bacterium can be cultured from the brain of affected pigs if a head from an untreated pig is submitted to a bacteriology laboratory, to confirm the diagnosis of streptococcal meningitis.

Infection in humans occurs when the dead pigs in this situation are subject to autopsy or dissection by workers who transfer blood from the affected pig into their own bloodstream, via unskilled knife cuts. Outbreaks and incidents of streptococcal infections in humans from this source occur globally, but are more prominent in areas with weaker regulations or knowledge surrounding disposal and consumption of farm pigs.

4.3b. Pigs affected with nervous signs can be given injections of a penicillin antibiotic and some sedation and placed into a quiet hospital-pen area. Many of these treated pigs can recover well.

There are no current vaccines that are effective for *S. suis*. Therefore strategic medication of weaner pigs is often needed to prevent damaging outbreaks. In-feed or in-water penicillin antibiotics are the most effective for this weaner medication programme. The occurrence of streptococcal meningitis is often associated with mixing of weaner pigs from different sources. Therefore the development of farm management systems that streamline groups of weaner pigs from one breeder farm source into a single nursery pig flow, with all-in, all-out management will generally reduce the number of cases of this common disease.

4.4   Case Study

The farmer operated a large breeder, nursery and finisher farm system, in a region with many other pig farms. The farm site had a variety of buildings for each phase of production. The breeder pigs and young piglets received an intermittent vaccination programme. The farmer sometimes purchased weaner and breeder pigs from other nearby farms, and placed them into the herd, to increase production numbers. The farmer noticed many depressed pigs and an increase in mortality in the nursery areas. Close inspection indicated that many pigs in these buildings were sick, dull and depressed, particularly the younger nursery pigs. Several of the older nursery and grower pigs that were 8–15 weeks old had developed nervous signs. These pigs were wandering and circling around and wobbling about when they walked, with odd gaits, including raising their legs in high steps and keeping their legs at a wide stance. Several pigs were also recumbent, some pigs had dull paralysis of their legs (Fig. 4.4.i) and others were trembling or had convulsions. At autopsy of some of these pigs, there were few changes noted, but there were some white speckles of necrosis of the tonsils area in the throat (Fig. 4.4ii).

Key Features

- Farm in pig-dense area.
- Nervous signs in grower pigs, including ataxia, paralysis and odd gaits.
- Many sick pigs in a group.

4.4a. What is this problem?
4.4b. What control measures may assist the herd?

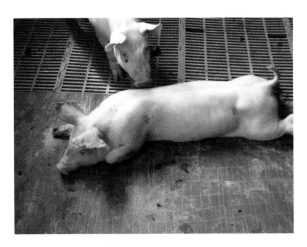

Fig. 4.4i. Weaner and grower pigs with paralysis and odd gaits.

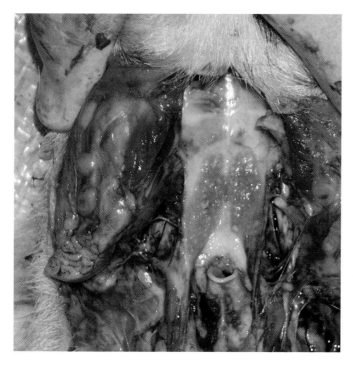

Fig. 4.4ii. Autopsy of affected nursery pig with white speckle necrosis in the throat.

4.4 Comments

4.4a. This type of herd problem with sick weaner pigs and odd nervous signs in grower pigs is suggestive of pseudorabies. This disease is due to a pig herpes virus. It is also known as Aujesky's disease in some countries. Outbreaks of disease are now less common, because of the widespread availability of useful vaccines and eradication programmes in some countries. However, in regions that remain positive for pseudorabies, it is a common disease of pigs, particularly in larger herds. It is often seen as a background problem on many farms, with occasional outbreaks of more severe illness and mortality. The virus is easily spread via pig-to-pig contact, so farms may experience more infections and problems when new pigs are introduced. In some pig farm areas, this new infection can occur when boars may be shared between farms, or when farms may purchase many pigs, as in this case study. When a pig is infected, the virus develops in the throat and can travel from there via the nerves into the brain, causing the nervous signs.

4.4b. Pseudorabies is generally controlled by the use of modern commercial vaccines. During an outbreak, the herd should be vaccinated and sick animals removed. This will lead to a recovery of the herd and may even eliminate the problem in the herd. There are various types of vaccine available, which can be given routinely to pigs in an infected herd. The repeated use of vaccines over some years can lead to full herd protection and elimination of clinical problems in small herds. However, in larger herds (more than 200 sows) the vaccines do not eliminate the disease, even when used for long periods.

4.5   Case Study

The farmer operated a newly constructed and modern breeder farm, with various lines of pig breeds (Fig. 4.5i). The new lines of breeder pigs and boars were purchased and used in various combinations for matings and pregnancy. The farrowing rates and numbers born alive were at the target levels. The farmer used a complete vaccination programme for the new breeding pigs. The farmer noticed that many young piglets in some litters were visibly shaking and trembling. Close inspection indicated that piglets in the affected litters were mainly from newly arrived gilts in pure-bred lines of Landrace or Saddleback pig matings (Fig. 4.5ii). The affected piglets continued to tremble and shake when standing and walking about. They had difficulty standing upright and difficulty getting to the teats. When the piglets were individually examined, it was noticed that they had tremors of the head, at 2–4 tremors/s. The tremors ceased when the piglets were sleeping. The pre-weaning mortality rates were increased in these litters, with some affected piglets suffering starvation or crushing. The mother gilts appeared normal. At autopsy of affected piglets, the brain, including the cerebellum area, appeared of normal size.

Key Features

- First few days after birth is the specific age range affected.
- Trembling and shaking when standing and walking.

4.5a. What is this problem?
4.5b. What control measures may assist the herd?

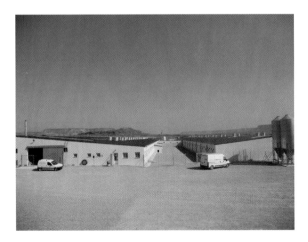

Fig. 4.5i. Newly constructed modern breeder farm in isolated area.

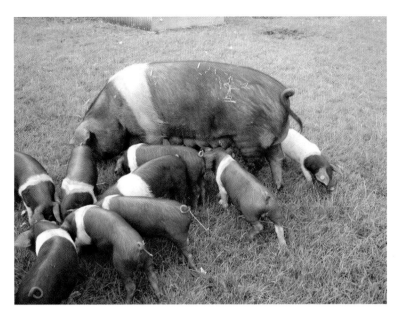

Fig. 4.5ii. Young Saddleback breed piglets with tremors.

4.5   Comments

4.5a. This condition is known as congenital tremors. The problem involves degeneration in the part of the piglet brain, known as the cerebellum, which is responsible for balance and muscle control. This problem can occur from two main causes: (i) it is inherited; or (ii) it is caused by mild virus infection.

The inherited form of congenital tremors is more common in some lines of pig breeds, particularly in Landrace or Saddleback pigs, so it will be noted in the piglets from specific combinations of matings. The most common type of inherited condition is probably in Landrace pure-bred matings, where the boar carries the genetic condition. In this form, the condition is mainly seen in male piglets. It is sometimes possible to view some tremors in the head and shoulders of the parent Landrace boars. Congenital tremors can also be seen in piglets from various combinations of Landrace, Saddleback and Large White pig breed matings.

The second form of congenital tremors occurs when a mild virus infection occurs in naïve gilts that have newly arrived at a breeder farm system. This virus infection causes the degeneration in the cerebellum in piglets, with the resulting tremors. In this form of tremors, a high proportion of piglets from these gilts will be affected.

4.5b. The affected piglets will often need assistance from farm workers to reach the teats and suckle colostrum in the first day of life. After suckling, these piglets can be removed and placed into a heated box area, to avoid crushing by the mother. The floors of the farrowing pens should have sufficient grip for small piglets to move around easily. This may involve the provision of rubber matting around the gilt in litters with the problem. In the inherited form of the condition, the matings and boar used for production of these piglets should be noted and avoided.

4.6   Case Study

The farmer operated an established farm system with breeder, nursery and finisher units, on a single site. The breeder pigs and young piglets all received a complete vaccination programme. The farm sites had a variety of older buildings, with pens in various stages of repair. Some of the farm buildings were damp and poorly heated. The farm had various health problems over the past years, including coughing and poor growth rates. The farmer also noticed that occasional grower and finisher pigs had developed a head tilt over the past few months (Fig. 4.6i). Close inspection indicated that only occasional pigs were affected, at various ages between 6 and 20 weeks old. The individual pigs placed their head continually on one angle, turned their head to the side and often walked in a circular direction (Fig. 4.6ii). These pigs would sometimes lose balance and fall over when walking in these circles. Treatment of the pigs with antibiotics did not produce major improvement in these signs.

Key Features

- Grower or older pig with distinctive head tilt.

4.6a. What is this problem?
4.6b. What control measures may assist the herd?

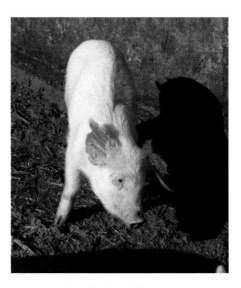

Fig. 4.6i. Individual young grower pig with head tilt.

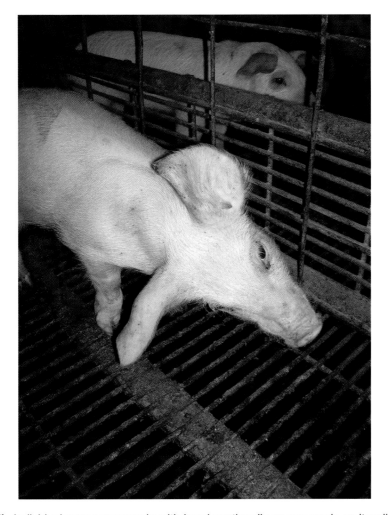

Fig. 4.6ii. Individual young grower pig with head continually on one angle so it walked in a circular direction.

4.6 Comments

4.6a. The signs of head tilt are suggestive of the condition known as a middle ear infection. This occurs where an infection enters the middle ear, setting up an ongoing abscess or nodule. The abscess presses painfully on to the brain near to the affected ear, causing the pig to lower the head on the affected side. The infection usually enters the middle ear via a tubular connection from the throat of the pig. Various bacteria may be associated with this lesion, such as Streptococcus. Middle ear infections are not a common problem in pig farms, with only occasional cases noted.

4.6b. Pigs often do not recover fully when treated, but may respond partially to penicillin injections. The middle ear area is not suitable for surgery in pigs. The problem is not common and so specific prevention measures are not usually necessary.

PART 5
Baby Piglet Problems

5.1 Case Study

The farmer operated an established medium-sized breeder farm, with various new and older buildings. These buildings had a mixture of older-style and new farrowing areas, with a variety of pen floors and devices for restraining the sows during the farrowing and lactation periods (Fig. 5.1i). The farmer employed a small number of staff to supervise the farrowings and piglet processing procedures in these areas. These staff also filled the feed troughs of the sows by hand in a morning rush-hour period. The farm had modern lines of pig breeds and the farrowing rate and numbers of piglets born alive were at the target levels. The farmer noticed that the pre-weaning mortality of young suckling piglets was consistently above 15% over a period of months. Close inspection of numerous litters over several weeks indicated that several pigs in each of the litters of neonatal piglets had become crushed and killed underneath the abdomen or legs of the sows (Fig. 5.1ii). Occasionally, a live piglet was discovered squealing loudly underneath a sow. Most of the affected piglets were 1–3 days of age. The worst affected litters and farrowing pens appeared to be those with fat sows in older-style farrowing areas on slippery floors.

Key Features

- Piglets in the first week of life crushed by the sow.

5.1a. What is this problem?
5.1b. What control measures may assist the herd?

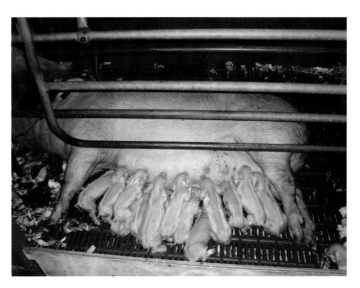

Fig. 5.1i. Fat sow in older-style farrowing-pen area.

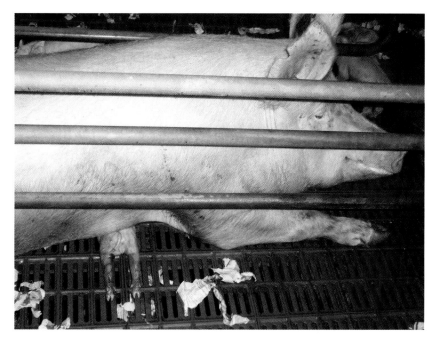

Fig. 5.1ii. Young piglet crushed under a sow.

5.1 Comments

5.1a. This is the common form of deaths due to crushing or overlay in piglets, as part of physical injury to the piglet by the sow. The widespread usage of metal crates or cradle devices that restrain the sow during farrowing and lactation, which were first adopted in the 1960s, lead to a marked reduction in this form of piglet death. However, even when farrowing crates are used, it can still be a common problem. Crushing is suggested to account for around 50% of all piglet deaths, usually in the first week of life. In farms that use open farrowing areas, without any form of sow restraint device, then piglet deaths due to crushing will be even higher. There are undoubtedly some sows that are clumsy and liable to wander about and flop down, without care for the piglets. These sows should be identified by farm records and culled. However, most cases are due to a variety of sow, piglet and environmental factors coming together in a farrowing area. The problem is often exacerbated by slippery floors in the lactation pens, which will make it difficult for the sow to lie down or get up easily. If the sows are too fat, then they are less active and more likely to drop to the ground suddenly, perhaps with a piglet underneath.

5.1b. The control of this common problem requires attention to the management of the farrowing and lactation areas. The sow needs to be matched to the size of the restraint device and pen area. Either too little or too much space will create opportunities for piglets to be crushed. The major disturbances caused when sows are fed manually by staff placing feed into troughs may lead to many excitable sows jumping up and down, with piglets underneath. Heating devices in lactation pens need to be carefully managed, to prevent piglets staying too close to the sow when they are sleeping and to allow the piglets to move around easily.

5.2 Case Study

The farmer operated an established medium-sized breeder farm, with modern lines of pig breeds. The farrowing rates and numbers born alive were at the target levels. The farmer used a complete vaccination programme for the breeding pigs. The farrowing and lactation areas were in older buildings, which had a low level of attention to the cleaning and hygiene for the floors, plastic-slat areas and pens (Fig. 5.2i). The farmer noticed that several litters had periods of moderate grey-to-yellow diarrhoea for periods of several days. Close inspection revealed that the affected piglets were generally 3–14 days old. The piglets had some grey-and-yellow faeces staining around their anus, with some loose faeces in the pens (Fig. 5.2ii), but the piglets were generally moving around and suckling well. There were a moderate number of litters affected; all the affected litters were from the first parity (gilt) pigs. These gilts appeared normal and the pre-weaning mortality rates were still within target levels. There was no response to antibiotic treatments to the piglets. At autopsy of some affected piglets, the farmer and veterinarian noticed that there was some dilation of the small intestines with soft liquid contents.

Key Features

- Piglets in first to third week of life.
- Mild forms of grey-to-yellow diarrhoea in piglets.

5.2a. What is this problem?
5.2b. What control measures may assist the herd?

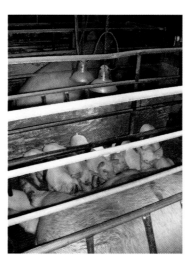

Fig. 5.2i. Older farrowing areas with low hygiene.

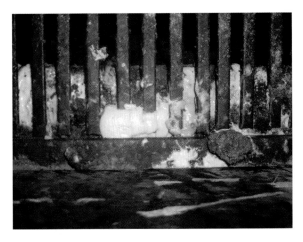

Fig. 5.2ii. Mild grey-to-yellow diarrhoea in suckling piglet pens.

5.2 Comments

5.2a. This type of moderate diarrhoea is likely to be the common form of rotavirus infection in pigs. This virus is a common infection on most pig farms. The virus is resistant in the environment and tends to build up over time, particularly in farrowing areas with poor hygiene. The piglets tend to pick up the virus from the environment and it will multiply in the small intestines and damage the villi. The mild clinical signs can make the actual diagnosis of rotavirus difficult. It may be confirmed by histopathology of the affected intestines that will demonstrate a mild-to-moderate villus atrophy consistent with rotavirus infection. Rotavirus may also be detected by PCR on intestinal contents. The affected litters are usually from gilts, because the levels of antibodies in a pig tend to build up over time. Older sows will pass on adequate maternal antibodies in their colostrum to prevent early infections in the piglets' intestines.

5.2b. There is no commercial vaccine or medication that is effective for rotavirus problems. So control measures will include nursing of affected piglets with extra warmth and nutrition.

Farrowing and lactation areas that are old and dirty will be a reservoir of rotavirus infection, if they are not cleaned properly. Cleaning of farrowing and lactation areas must include the initial use of detergents to remove the fatty and grease-filled areas derived from sow milk, prior to washing and use of disinfectants. In farrowing areas with plastic slats, these need to be lifted from the pens and cleaned and washed in the detergents and disinfectants. The farrowing pens should be rested between litters for as long as possible. The amount of faecal material (slurry) underneath farrowing and lactation pens needs to be managed properly.

Some authorities recommend the procedure of feeding faecal materials to the gilts in late gestation. This faecal material may be diarrhoea from the affected piglets collected on toilet paper. This paper can then be fed twice a week to the gilts for the last 4 weeks of their pregnancy. This exposure to diarrhoea rotavirus (and other agents) gives the gilt the chance to develop some immunity and increase the amount of their antibodies to the virus. The gilt will then hopefully pass on these antibodies to the piglets and lead to a reduction in the overall problem.

5.3 Case Study

The farmer operated an established medium-sized breeder farm, with modern lines of pig breeds. The farrowing rates and numbers born alive were generally at the target levels. The farmer did not use a complete vaccination programme for the breeding pigs. The farrowing and lactation areas were in older buildings, which were used for an increasing number of farrowing sows. The farm had a low level of attention to the cleaning and hygiene for the floors, plastic-slat areas and pens. The farmer noticed that all of the piglets in several litters had periods of explosive white-to-yellow–orange diarrhoea. The farm workers stated that the piglets were 'born with diarrhoea'. The problem seemed to be spreading around the farrowing and lactation areas. Close inspection revealed that the affected piglets were generally young, at 1–7 days old. They had watery diarrhoea, which was ejected as a stream from the anus (Fig. 5.3i). The piglets were depressed, huddling together and not moving around (Fig. 5.3ii). The pre-weaning mortality rates were rising above target levels and the weights of piglets at weaning were low. There were many litters affected with the diarrhoea problem, and all these litters were from the first parity (gilt) pigs. These gilts appeared normal. There appeared to be some response to antibiotic treatments of the piglets. At autopsy of some affected piglets, there was marked dehydration of the body and loss of fat reserves, with marked dilation of the small and large intestines with watery yellow-liquid contents. The stomach contained plenty of milk and there was a reddening congestion of the lining of the stomach wall.

Key Features

- Litters of young piglets from non-vaccinated gilts affected.
- Yellow watery diarrhoea faeces.

5.3a. What is this problem?
5.3b. What control measures may assist the herd?

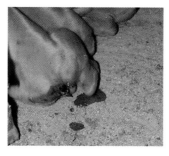

Fig. 5.3i. Young piglets with watery diarrhoea.

5.3 Comments

5.3a. The findings of watery diarrhoea in many young piglets from gilt litters is suggestive of the common form of neonatal colibacillosis in piglets. The bacteria that cause neonatal colibacillosis are enterotoxigenic strains of *Escherichia coli* (ETEC). These bacteria are located in the farrowing-pen environment and are ingested by the piglet soon after birth. The bacteria then attach to the small intes-

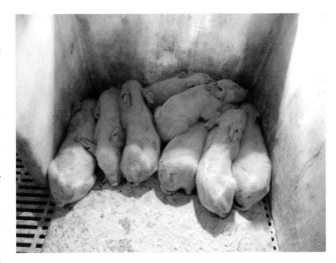

Fig. 5.3ii. Sick young piglets in older farrowing area.

tine and cause an outpouring of fluid into the intestine and watery diarrhoea. In some cases, the sick piglets can resemble piglets that have failed to take in much milk, for example if the gilt did not produce sufficient milk. The ETEC can be cultured in a bacteriology laboratory from the watery contents of the small intestine. It is important to collect intestine contents material at the autopsy of a fresh piglet for this test – the simple collection of faeces from cases of diarrhoea in piglets will not lead to a successful culture or diagnosis. Neonatal colibacillosis is a common cause of loss in piglets soon after birth, but it has become less common because of the availability of effective commercial vaccines that can be given to gilts and sows on the breeder farm.

5.3b. Individual litters and piglets may be treated with oral antibiotics, which must be given to the entire litter at the earliest sign of diarrhoea. The treatment of piglets must also provide rehydration electrolytes. These are to replace the body fluids that are quickly lost in the diarrhoea episodes in small piglets. These electrolytes may be given by a clean syringe into the mouth or rectum of each piglet. It is important to attempt to limit the spread of the ETEC around the farrowing rooms. Handling of affected piglets should be done after normal ones are handled. Separate boots and clothes may be used for an infected area, with clean ones provided for other areas. Piglets should remain in the infected area and not moved to other sows. The udders of affected gilts and sows should be washed and cleaned regularly.

Vaccines against ETEC are widely available and are best given to the gilts and sows to raise systemic immunity and antibody levels, which then appear in the colostrum and are transferred to piglets, providing protection from the ETEC infection in the piglets.

Farrowing and lactation areas that are old and dirty will be a reservoir of ETEC infection, if they are not cleaned properly. Cleaning of farrowing and lactation areas must include the initial use of detergents to remove the fatty and grease-filled areas derived from sow milk, prior to washing and use of disinfectants. The farrowing pens should be rested and kept dry between litters for as long as possible.

5.4 Case Study

The farmer operated a medium-sized breeding farm, with many sows kept in outdoor pen areas for gestation, farrowing and lactation stages (Fig. 5.4i). These outdoor pens had a variety of feeder and water stations and shelters for the sows and piglets. The breeder pigs were developed with modern lines of pig breeds, which were adapted to outdoor breeding techniques. The breeder gilts and sows were vaccinated against *E. coli*, erysipelas and parvovirus. The farrowing rates and numbers born alive were at the target levels. The farmer noticed that some litters suffered many sudden deaths of young piglets and other litters had several small, runt piglets with some diarrhoea. Close inspection indicated that the affected litters were mainly derived from gilts. In 20–30% of litters there were sporadic cases of deaths, poor growth and diarrhoea in these piglets, mainly in the first week of life. The runt piglets were thin, sunken eyed and dehydrated. Some of these piglets had a red anus, and watery, dark bloody-brown diarrhoea (Fig. 5.4ii). At autopsy of some these piglets, the middle of the small intestine (jejunum) appeared very dark and intensely congested red to a fire-engine red colour, with some gas and bloody fluid present. The lymph nodes around the intestines were dark and haemorrhagic. In some piglets, the reaction consisted more of soft thickening with fluid in the intestine wall and necrotic areas on the mucosal lining.

Key Features

- Piglets in the first week of life on an outdoor breeder pig farm.
- Bloody diarrhoea faeces and intestines.

5.4a. What is this problem?
5.4b. What control measures may assist the herd?

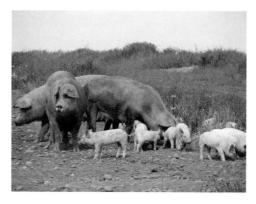

Fig. 5.4i. Young piglets in outdoor breeding herd.

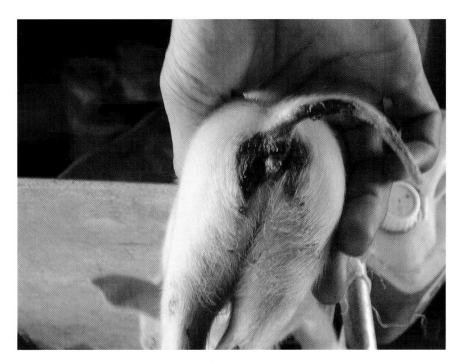

Fig. 5.4ii. Piglet with dark bloody-brown diarrhoea.

5.4   Comments

5.4a. This type of bloody diarrhoea and deaths in piglets is suggestive of infections with the Clostridia bacteria. These are a group of bacteria that normally reside in the soil and faeces. *Clostridium perfringens* is one of the causative species in this group, but other Clostridia may also be involved in this suckling-pig diarrhoea problem. This problem mainly occurs in areas of outdoor breeding farms where the soil is contaminated and the piglets can access this material. These bacteria attach to the piglet intestines and possess potent toxins, which cause necrosis and bloody outflow in the intestines. This Clostridia problem is rarely seen in indoor farms, but may become apparent where piglets are injected with antibiotics that eliminate other bacteria and allow the Clostridia to become a dominant strain.

5.4b. Clostridia are fully susceptible to penicillin antibiotics; therefore the piglets born in outdoor farms may be treated soon after birth with long-acting amoxicillin. It is important to keep lactation sows clean of soil and faeces where possible. Some commercial vaccines now exist for the control of *C. perfringens* in pigs. Breeder pigs in outdoor herds should be given a full vaccine schedule with these vaccines in addition to the other breeder vaccines. Breeder pigs in indoor herds can also be vaccinated if the problem has been noticed in the herd.

In contrast to the notes on feeding faecal materials to gilts in the last 4 weeks of their pregnancy, which were mentioned in other case studies (e.g. see Case Study 5.2), the experience is that providing this material where Clostridia disease occurs will make the situation worse. The feedback material will increase the amount of the Clostridia bacteria in the farrowing gilt environment and increase the dose to piglets.

5.5 Case Study

The farmer operated an established medium-sized breeder farm, with various older-style buildings. The farrowing and lactation pens were in smaller closed rooms in older buildings, with small windows and low roofs. The farrowing rates with modern lines of pig breeds were at the target levels. The farmer used a complete vaccination programme for the breeding pigs. During long periods of cold weather, the farmer used a variety of old gas heaters to heat these small farrowing rooms (Fig. 5.5i). During one period of very cold weather, the farmer noticed that several litters had many piglets born dead or dying in the first few days of life. Close inspection indicated that the entire litter was affected, with all the piglets in the litter found dead. The piglets in these cases of stillbirths and neonatal deaths were not a normal colour; the affected piglets had a bright cherry-red skin colour (Fig. 5.5ii). An inspection of the room heaters indicated that some of the old ones were not adjusted properly and were producing yellow flames (not the normal blue flame). There was no abnormal odour or taste in the rooms.

Key Features

- Small closed farrowing rooms with gas flame heaters.
- Stillbirths and deaths of piglets in the first week of life.

5.5a. What is this problem?
5.5b. What control measures may assist the herd?

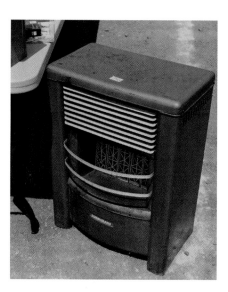

Fig. 5.5i. Gas flame heater used to heat older buildings.

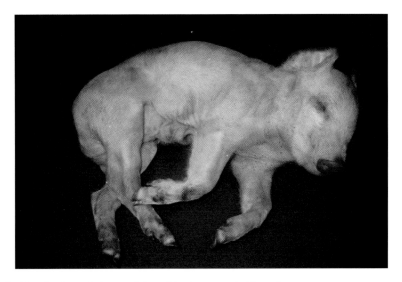

Fig. 5.5ii. Death of newly born piglet with cherry-red skin colour.

5.5 Comments

5.5a. This condition is the common form of carbon monoxide (CO) gas poisoning. This is a relatively common occurrence on small indoor pig farms in cold weather, where gas heaters are used. The fatal poisoning usually occurs when poorly adjusted or damaged gas-burning heaters are operated in small spaces, such as poorly ventilated farrowing houses. When CO gas levels go above 250 ppm in the room atmosphere, then litters of baby piglets may be found dead, or groups of late pregnant sows within the affected building area may give birth to entire litters of dead piglets.

5.5b. The safety and prosperity of the pigs and people on a pig farm are the first priority of any such enterprise. The placement and raising of domestic pigs into housed, indoor or outdoor accommodation creates a strong and specific responsibility for attendants and managers to take care of every need of their pigs and prevent any mishandling of them. Work instructions, often known as a standard operating procedure (SOP) should be prepared for each task identified in each area of the farm and displayed at the place where the work is to be carried out. These instructions specify the actual steps to be taken to safely perform a task, such as: (i) the use of heaters; (ii) proper ventilation; (iii) the administration of vaccines; or (iv) operation of a farm vehicle. A separate record should be kept of the safe systems of work related to each of these procedures. This document should include: (i) general safety points; (ii) the general code of practice for all workers; and (iii) a risk assessment of the nature of any particular hazard (such as gas heaters or noisy squealing pigs). These records and SOPs should be prepared for all normal operations and available for inspection by any technical visitor, or in any legal situation, following an accident.

Besides the CO poisoning illustrated in this case study, other poisons on pig farms include poisonous chemicals such as rodent poisons, crop and livestock chemicals, such as organophosphates, used for pest and insect control. It is vital to properly label these toxic chemicals and exclude all of them from around any feed preparation or mixing operation.

5.6   Case Study

The farmer operated a medium-sized breeder farm, with modern lines of pig breeds. The farrowing rates and numbers born alive were at the target levels. The farmer used a complete vaccination programme for the breeding pigs. The farm was located in an area with many other farms in the region. Trucks moved between these farms for feed delivery and collection of dead pigs and dead piglets. A few days after some dirty trucks had entered the farm, the farmer noticed a rapidly spreading outbreak of diarrhoea among numerous litters of piglets in the farrowing and lactation rooms. Close inspection indicated a high proportion of the litters were all affected simultaneously, at ages of 2–4 weeks old. The affected piglets had large amounts of watery to soft yellow-to-green diarrhoea (Fig. 5.6i), with many piglets also seen to be vomiting yellow milky fluids. The piglets were dull and not suckling well. The piglets did not respond to antibiotic treatments, but appeared to slowly recover after being sick for 1 week. At autopsy of sick piglets, the farmer and veterinarian noticed the small intestine was distended with watery yellow fluid (Fig. 5.6ii). The mucosal lining of the intestines appeared thin. Over the following weeks, the pre-weaning mortality levels were markedly increased above normal levels.

Key Features

- Outbreaks of yellow watery diarrhoea faeces in piglets.
- Small intestines distended with yellow watery fluid.

5.6a. What is this problem?

5.6b. What control measures may assist the herd?

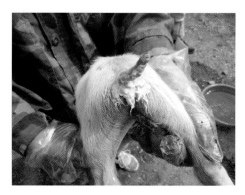

Fig. 5.6i. Yellow watery to soft diarrhoea in piglets from affected pens.

5.6 Comments

5.6a. This type of spectacular outbreak of yellow watery diarrhoea in piglets is the common form of PED. It is caused by a pig coronavirus. There are a group of related coronaviruses in pigs around the world, which cause very similar forms of this disease, including viruses known as TGE and HEV. At the moment, PED is the most common and important form of pig coronavirus disease, with recent spread

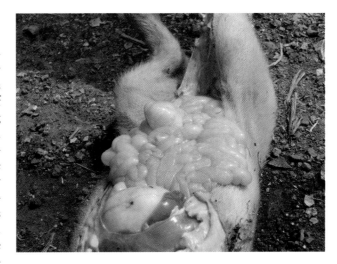

Fig. 5.6ii. Small intestines distended with yellow watery fluid.

around many pig farming regions globally. The experience in current PED outbreaks is that breakdowns occur on many farms every 6–12 months. Outbreaks of PED can vary in intensity and duration, sometimes with many older pigs affected also. The diagnosis of PED can be confirmed by blood tests or PCR tests. The high level of pre-weaning mortality will have obvious consequences on production. However, it also appears that PED can have long-term effects on sow performance. The subsequent litter size will drop due to the shorter lactation lengths because of the PED piglet mortality, with irregular returns to oestrus.

5.6b. Sick piglets may be fed with milk substitute products and provided with warmth while they are nursed to recovery. The treatment of piglets must also provide rehydration electrolytes. These are to replace the body fluids that are quickly lost in the vomiting and diarrhoea episodes in small piglets.

The main method for limiting the duration of an outbreak of PED remains the use of a controlled exposure of the breeder pigs to live PED virus-positive material. This acts to enhance natural immunity of the breeder herd and increase maternal antibodies in the sow colostrum, so providing some protection to the piglets. The usual advice for the best chances of getting feedback to work requires: (i) to get as much affected piglet material (intestines) as possible; (ii) homogenize it; (iii) put some antibiotics into it to kill any Salmonella bacteria; and (iv) feed it to the entire breeding herd. Control of outbreaks on problem farms remains largely an attempt to raise herd immunity by use of live virus feedback material derived from affected piglet intestines. The most successful programmes are therefore usually when the sows and gilts are exposed several times to the feedback material. Exposing the sows and gilts may also result in depression, apathy and anorexia and abortions.

A number of local attenuated and killed vaccines for PED are available. The actual usefulness of these various PED vaccines on problem farms has probably been very limited.

The control of PED on farms also requires reduction of rodent and bird populations and restriction of their entry to farms and feed areas. Great care and attention must be paid to cleaning any trucks that enter the farm, particularly those that may be carrying or collecting pigs.

5.7 Case Study

The farmer operated a modern breeder farm, with new lines of commercial pig breeds. The farrowing rates and numbers born alive were at the target levels. The farmer used a complete vaccination programme for the breeding pigs. The new lines of breeder pigs were moved around between different buildings, with various groups and sizes of pigs in large and small pens. In one breeding-pig group of Large White breed pigs, the gilts in their first gestation were raised in large group sizes, of 50–100 pigs, in large, open pens (Fig. 5.7i). These pigs were then moved in late pregnancy to their individual farrowing pens. The farmer noticed that many of these gilts appeared nervous and were seen to attack their newly born piglets. Close inspection indicated that these gilts had a wild-eyed and crazy look, and showed apprehensive fear responses in the farrowing pens and to the farm workers. Following the birth process, many of the young piglets in these litters appeared normal but were attacked by the gilt and the piglets had bite wounds and teeth injuries around their body (Fig. 5.7ii). Several piglet deaths occurred due to these attacks, causing a rise in pre-weaning mortality.

Key Features

- Litters from nervous gilts in modern pig lines.
- Bite wounds and injuries in newborn piglets.

5.7a. What is this problem?
5.7b. What control measures may assist the herd?

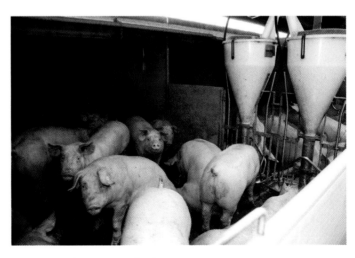

Fig. 5.7i. Large groups of pregnant gilts in pens.

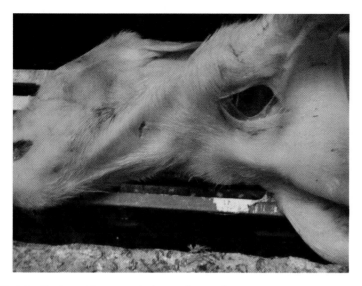

Fig. 5.7ii. Piglet with deep bite wounds from gilt attack.

5.7 Comments

5.7a. This problem is known as gilt savaging and refers to the first-parity mother gilt attacking her newly born offspring. It occurs occasionally in many animal species, when giving birth for the first time. It may be related to the hormonal changes and high pain levels that occur at this stage of the female's life. In pigs, it is seen more often with specific forms of pig flow in harsh environments, such as large groups of boisterous or aggressive gilts, which are suddenly moved to a farrowing-pen environment, as suggested in this case study. In these large groups of gilts, no social order develops and each gilt must nervously consider all others as an enemy, including their own offspring. Some other factors seem to occur in many of these outbreaks, such as poorly trained farm staff, dietary changes, and in specific lines and breeds of Large White pigs, which may have a more nervous temperament.

5.7b. Any gilt giving birth must be observed carefully for signs of nervousness and savaging. When the gilt remains nervous and restless with her newly born litter, so she does not lie down and relax, then she may require a tranquilliser or sedative. Unfortunately, no simple, universal, quick and safe sedative exists for pigs. The sedative, azaperone (often marketed as Stresnil®) can be given as an intramuscular injection dose. Alternatively, the sedative acepromazine can be given as an intramuscular injection dose or as an oral dose of 3 ml per gilt. The piglets are kept aside for 20–30 min after the sedative has been given to the gilt, then are reintroduced. This procedure can act to settle individual gilts and the lactation of the litter can proceed normally. If neither of these sedatives is available, then large cans of beer can be provided to the gilt (not to the farmer). Late pregnant gilts should be placed into stalls or individual pig pens for 1 week prior to farrowing and housed next to farrowing sows. The farrowing-room environment should be dark and warm, with caring staff attending to the gilts. If a gilt appears to be wild-eyed, then a young piglet can be placed in her pen prior to her farrowing, to test her reaction.

5.8 Case Study

The farmer operated a modern breeder farm, with some new lines of commercial pig breeds. The new lines of breeder pigs and boars were shifted in various combinations for matings and pregnancy. The farrowing rates and numbers born alive were at the target levels. The farmer used a complete vaccination programme for the breeding pigs. Litters of pigs were generally raised for eventual sale as finisher pigs. To prevent the undesirable male-related traits in pigs, namely aggressive pubertal behaviour traits and the obnoxious boar taint smell and taste arising in the pork and fat of entire male pigs, all male pigs were physically castrated at 3 days of age. The farm workers made a short open cut above each testicle and the entire testicle and epididymis were removed (Fig. 5.8i). The farm workers then noticed that during this castration process, some piglets appeared to have portions of their intestines mixed in with the testicles. Close inspection indicated that these piglets had portions of intestines protruding through an inguinal hernia in the abdomen into the scrotum, particularly on the left side (Fig. 5.8ii). They were derived from matings with one line of boars. The farmer mentioned that some of these hernia pigs had been ignored and had gone through to finisher pig stage. The farmer and his staff had also attempted some surgical procedures on the male piglets with hernias, during the castration process. Some of these surgery piglets had then developed severe ulcers with bloody fluids and smelly necrotic skin around the scrotum area.

Key Features

- Male piglets with inguinal hernia and intestines entering the scrotum.

5.8a. What are these problems?
5.8b. What control measures may assist the herd?

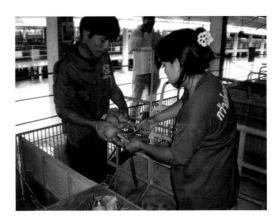

Fig. 5.8i. Processing and surgery of male piglets.

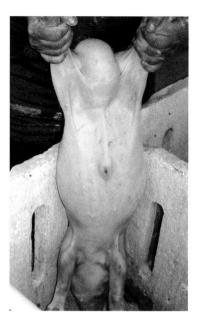

Fig. 5.8ii. Hernia with intestines entering into the scrotum of a male piglet.

5.8 Comments

5.8a. The condition where intestines enter the scrotum in male piglets is the common form of inguinal or scrotal hernia. It is a common inherited defect of pigs, with a suggested incidence of up to 1% of piglets. The hernia may be noticed when the piglet is being castrated and the intestines appear in the scrotal area. In this case repair is very difficult. However, pigs with scrotal hernias can be identified by holding them upside down by the hind legs and squeezing their abdomen. If a bulge appears in either inguinal area, that pig has a scrotal hernia and should not be castrated in the normal fashion. It may also be noticed when the finisher pig goes to slaughter, and this will result in the carcass being downgraded. The use of inappropriate surgery on the scrotum can lead to the cases of severe local infections known as inguinal cellulitis, with large ulcerative cysts and necrotic skin lesions over the scrotum area. This lesion is seen if the surgery is performed with the wrong type of suture materials that are non-absorbable or vinyl suture materials.

A range of other inherited defects occur in pigs and are described in other cases.
5.8b. Inguinal or scrotal hernias can only be fixed by proper surgery, prior to any routine castration. The correct open surgical repair of inguinal hernia in male piglets basically requires that the testicle area is opened and the testicle tunic is twisted and sutured while twisted, so that the intestinal contents are returned to the abdomen and held there. Examples of this technique in use in pigs are available in video format at the YouTube website. The use of sharp and clean specialized scalpel instruments, antiseptic hygiene, wound dressing and staff training is vital for routine castrations and this repair procedure. The use of anaesthetic substances (local or general) during routine castrations or this procedure is controversial, as these substances can be dangerous for farm workers during routine farm usage.

5.9   Case Study

The farmer operated an established medium-sized breeder farm, with modern lines of pig breeds. The farrowing rates and numbers born alive were generally at the target levels. The farmer used a complete vaccination programme for the breeding pigs. The farrowing and lactation areas were in older buildings, which were used for an increasing number of farrowing sows. The farm had a low level of attention to the cleaning and hygiene for the floors, plastic-slatted floor areas and pens. The farmer noticed that the numbers of deaths among pre-weaning piglets was increasing. Close inspection indicated that the deaths were mainly occurring in litters of young piglets derived from gilts, in the first few days after birth. Several of these young piglets were noticed to be dull and walking in a weak manner. These piglets appeared cold, shivering, with poor breathing and blue extremities. These piglets did not eat readily, and were generally huddled in groups in the farrowing areas (Fig. 5.9i). Many piglets died soon after it was noticed they were sick (Fig. 5.9ii). The mother sows had adequate milk production and other litters of older piglets appeared normal. At autopsy of the affected young piglets, the stomach was empty and the internal organs appeared slightly dark and congested. There was no clear evidence of diarrhoea or other specific sign.

Key Features

- Illness and deaths among piglets in the first week of life.
- Apparent failure of colostrum intake.

5.9a. What is this problem?
5.9b. What control measures may assist the herd?

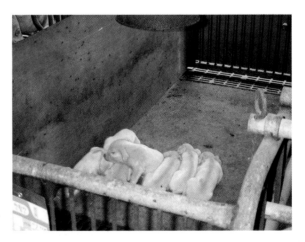

Fig. 5.9i. Sick young piglets huddle in groups.

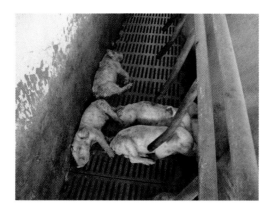

Fig. 5.9ii. Deaths of young piglets.

5.9 Comments

5.9a. This condition is the common form of *Escherichia coli* septicaemia in young piglets, known as coli-septicaemia. The *E. coli* bacterium can be grown in pure culture from the internal organs of these cases, in a bacteriology laboratory, to confirm the diagnosis. These cases occur when there is insufficient intake of colostrum by the newly born piglets. This leads to an insufficient intake and transfer of colostrum antibody to the piglets and a reduction in their blood levels of antibodies (known as hypogammaglobulinaemia) needed to fight the bacteria in their new environment. Unlike in dogs and humans, there is no transfer of any protective materials through the placental membranes in foetal pigs. The piglet is therefore born 'naked' and requires an immediate intake of these protective materials, such as cells and antibodies, contained in the first milk of the sow, or colostrum. The colostrum should be yellow, sticky and creamy and produced for the first day of lactation. *E. coli* are common bacteria in the environment and the problem may be more common on farms that have a busy number of farrowings and have poor hygiene, leading to a high level of *E. coli* bacteria embedded in the dirty pens. This case study of coli-septicaemia can be similar in presentation and causative factors, to cases of low milk production or agalactia in sows. Coli-septicaemia may also be seen in conjunction with cases of mastitis in sows.

5.9b. The management of the farrowing areas requires high quality staff, who are caring and pay attention to the needs of newborn piglets, to suckle well and acquire colostrum. There should be sufficient staff to adequately monitor newborn litters, including those born at night-time. Individual affected piglets may be treated with antibiotics and pig gamma-globulin injections. The udders of affected gilts and sows should be washed and cleaned regularly. Vaccines against *E. coli* are widely available and are given to the gilts and sows to raise systemic immunity in late pregnancy, which then appears in the colostrum and is transferred to the piglets.

Farrowing and lactation areas that are old and dirty will be a reservoir of infection, if they are not cleaned properly. Cleaning of farrowing and lactation areas must include the initial use of detergents to remove the fatty and grease-filled areas derived from sow milk, prior to washing and use of disinfectants. The farrowing pens should be rested and kept dry between litters for as long as possible. The amount of faeces material (slurry) underneath farrowing and lactation pens needs to be managed properly.

5.10   Case Study

The farmer operated a medium-sized breeder farm, with modern lines of pig breeds. The farrowing rate and numbers of pigs born alive were at the target levels. The breeding programme had improved the litter size, with most litters now having 11 or more piglets. The farrowing pens were in modern well-constructed buildings. The farmer tended to move piglets around between litters to assist the management of even litter sizes. The farmer noticed that the pre-weaning mortality of piglets in the larger litters had increased from 10% to 12% and several suckling piglets were noticed to have rough skin patches on the side of their faces. Close inspection indicated that the affected piglets were 2–7 days old with crusty, dark, roughened patches and scabs of necrotic skin on their facial cheeks. Many piglets in these litters also had sharp needle teeth, which appeared to protrude sideways in some piglets (Fig. 5.10i). Piglets from both sows and gilts were affected. Some of the sows also had areas of injuries around the teats. The more severely affected piglets had larger lesions on their cheeks (Fig. 5.10ii) and were reluctant to suckle, with a loss of body condition. These severe lesions tended to heal slowly, taking a few weeks to heal, even with antibiotic administration.

Key Features

- Piglets in first week of life with necrotic facial lesions.

5.10a. What is this problem?
5.10b. What control measures may assist the herd?

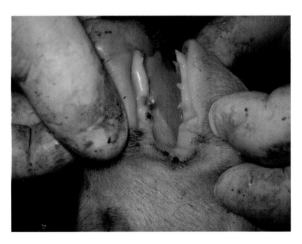

Fig. 5.10i. Sharp protruding needle teeth in piglet.

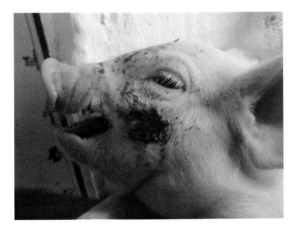

Fig. 5.10ii. Dark crusty lesion on the face and cheeks of a piglet.

5.10 Comments

5.10a. This condition with injuries and infections of the face in piglets is known as facial necrosis. It is a common problem on many pig farms around the world. The pointy, sharp third (corner) incisor and canine (needle teeth) are usually present at birth of piglets. In many piglets, these teeth can protrude from the side of the mouth. In large active litters, the competition for teats can lead to aggression between piglets, with facial injuries inflicted on cohort piglets by these teeth. Secondary infection of these facial injuries is also common, usually with bacteria such as staphylococci and anaerobes, leading to the messy, dark necrotic lesions. Facial necrosis is very common where the management of lactation and litters leads to a lot of piglet movement between litters. These relocated piglets tend to fight among each other to reclaim a nursing spot on a teat. Facial necrosis can lead to a significant increase in pre-weaning mortality. The sharp needle teeth in large litters can also lead to teat injuries and reduced milk production in the sows. This important problem is the reason for the preventative practice of clipping of needle teeth in baby piglets, on many farms.

5.10b. For each affected piglet, the face should be washed and cleaned and the piglet given a penicillin antibiotic by injection and on to the facial lesions directly. While healing of minor lesions can occur in a few days, piglets with more severe lesions can take 2–3 weeks to heal, even with the use of antibiotics.

Routine teeth clipping can be carried out within the first day of life, but not before 6 h of age. Alternatively, teeth clipping may be performed at 2–3 days old, when facial damage is being noted. Teeth clipping may also be limited to those litters where piglets have been added. Trimming consists of clipping or grinding the protruding canine teeth, to the level of the gums. Properly trained staff and the use of sharp and clean specialized clipper instruments are vital. Transitory pain will occur, but piglets are usually observed to suckle almost immediately after clipping has occurred. If clipping is rushed, or poor quality instruments are used, then the clipped teeth will shatter, leading to local infections. Teeth-clipping instruments must be separate from tail-cutting instruments.

Reducing the movement of pigs between litters leads to reduced fighting and consequently reduced facial necrosis.

5.11   Case Study

The farmer operated an established medium-sized breeder farm, with modern lines of pig breeds. The farrowing rates and numbers born alive were at the target levels. The farmer used a complete vaccination programme for the breeding pigs. The farrowing and lactation areas were in older buildings, which had old and draughty windows over the pens. The breeder farm had an increasing number of farrowing sows, with many placed into these older buildings and farrowing pens. There were only a few heaters available and few mats or covers for the bare and damp floors of the farrowing pens (Fig. 5.11i). Several of the water points were old and dripped water around these pens. During the first month of colder winter weather, the farmer noticed that the pre-weaning mortality increased above 12%. Close inspection indicated that many young piglets less than 1 week old were weak, slow moving and tended to huddle in groups, often near to the sow's udder (Fig. 5.11ii). The piglets were interested in the sow udder, but did not suckle often. The piglets were cold to the touch and the floors of the farrowing pens were also cold and damp. Some piglets lay on their side with some twitching and died in a dull coma.

Key Features

- Newborn piglets in cold and damp farrowing pens.

5.11a. What is this problem?
5.11b. What control measures may assist the herd?

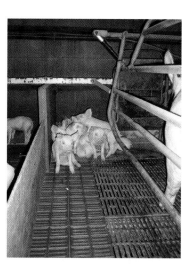

Fig. 5.11i. Piglets in cold and damp farrowing pens with no heating.

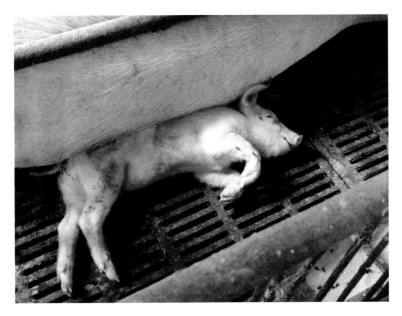

Fig. 5.11ii. Weak and chilled piglet huddled near to the sow.

5.11 Comments

5.11a. These are deaths of young piglets due to hypothermia or chilling. Piglets are born out of the warm environment of the uterus directly into the cold and wet environment of the farrowing area. Newly born piglets do not have much innate heat capacity or energy reserves. Therefore the management of farrowing rooms in breeding farms needs to provide adequate heating, with a room temperature of 20°C and a brighter section within the lactation pens, which is further heated to at least 35°C, to provide a safe and warm space for the piglets to sleep away from the sow. The piglets also need to suckle milk and colostrum rapidly to provide nutrition to generate their own body heat. Piglet chilling will occur if the farrowing pens are draughty and the floors are cold and damp, with inadequate dry mats, and the sleeping areas are not adequately heated. When piglets become chilled, they will move towards the sow to try to stay warm and may suffer more from crushing injury. Chilling is therefore likely to be a factor in crushing injuries, if many of the crushed piglets are noticed to have empty stomachs.

5.11b. The farrowing areas need to have adequate building maintenance with an absence of door, curtain and window draughts, with pens containing suitable sleeping areas, active heat lamps and warm, dry floors. This is particularly important in regions with cold weather periods. Many farms use some bedding materials and mats to assist the piglets find a warm and dry sleeping area. Farrowing pens need to be given adequate time to be dried after cleaning, between lactation periods. Chilling is a common problem on many farms with poor management of the farrowing rooms. The numbers of staff, staff training and attention to the many details of caring for young piglets need to be addressed, for the target level of 10% pre-weaning mortality to be regularly achieved.

5.12   Case Study

The farmer operated an established breeder farm, with modern lines of pig breeds. The farrowing rates and numbers born alive were at the target levels. The farmer used a complete vaccination programme for the breeding pigs. The farrowing and lactation rooms were in older buildings, with concrete floors and some wooden constructions. During the hotter and warmer months, the farmer noticed that several litters of suckling piglets had periods of diarrhoea. Close inspection indicated that most affected piglets were 1–2 weeks old and appeared thin with a poor body condition. Affected piglets had grey-to-yellow faeces that were soft, creamy and pasty, resembling toothpaste (Fig. 5.12i). Piglets in litters from both sows and gilts were affected. The mothers appeared normal and the piglets were drinking milk normally. There was a reduction in weaning weights of the piglets, with some increase in pre-weaning mortality. The diarrhoea problem did not respond to antibiotics. At autopsy of some affected piglets, the intestines had pasty-to-liquid contents and a pale, chalk-like appearance to the inner mucosal surface of the middle of the small intestine. Samples of the intestine were processed in a laboratory for histology and close examination of the epithelial cells of the small intestine revealed damage associated with the presence of banana-shape coccidian forms (Fig. 5.12ii).

Key Features

- Piglets in second week of life.
- Yellow–grey toothpaste-like faeces.

5.12a. What is this problem?
5.12b. What control measures may assist the herd?

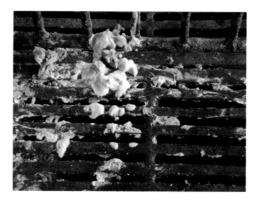

Fig. 5.12i. Ten-day-old piglet pens with yellow–grey toothpaste-like faeces.

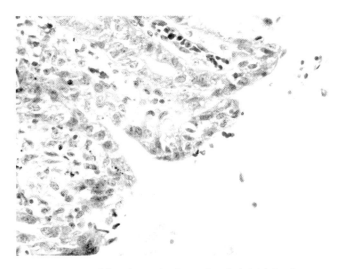

Fig. 5.12ii. Banana-shape coccidian forms in the cells of piglet intestine.

5.12 Comments

5.12a. This condition is the common form of coccidiosis in pigs, caused by a parasite known as *Isospora suis*. It usually occurs in the second week of life of the piglets. It is a common problem on many breeder pig farms around the world. Coccidia are small microscopic parasites that pass eggs (known as oocysts) in the piglet faeces and these oocysts stay on the floor of the farrowing pens. The oocysts develop into infective stages in the environment, provided the temperature exceeds 16°C. The piglets in the same litter or the next litter in the contaminated pen will take in these oocysts shortly after birth. *I. suis* then develops in the cells of the intestines of piglets over several days and causes damage to the lining of the intestine, often by the time the piglets are around 2 weeks old. The disease is often worse in warmer weather, when oocysts survive better in the pens. Confirmation of the disease is best done by recognition of the coccidian forms in the intestines. Coccidiosis problems will have a major negative effect on overall weaning weights and increase the number of days for infected pigs to eventually reach slaughter weights.

5.12b. Individual litters and piglets affected with coccidiosis may be treated with oral antibiotics of the sulfonamide/trimethoprim category. The treatment of piglets should also provide rehydration electrolytes. These are to replace the body fluids that are lost in the diarrhoea episodes of the piglets. These electrolytes may be given by a clean syringe into the mouth or rectum of each piglet. No piglet vaccines are available. Therefore for prevention, the potent anticoccidial drug toltrazuril is recommended as a single oral dose at 3–4 days old, to disrupt the life cycle of the parasite.

Efforts should be made to sterilize the floors of farrowing pens. This is difficult on many types of floors, including old concrete or wooden floors or plastic slats and many farrowing pens carry long-term infections with coccidial oocysts. The oocysts are very resistant to conventional disinfectants. Effective treatments are fire (flame gun) or washing the pens with lime. Another alternative is to paint the floors of the farrowing pens – the paint covers over the coccidiosis oocysts.

5.13   Case Study

The farmer operated a modern breeder farm, with various lines of pig breeds. The new lines of breeder pigs and boars were used in various combinations for matings and pregnancy. The farrowing rates and numbers of piglets born alive were at the target levels. The farmer used a complete vaccination programme for the breeding pigs. The farmer noticed that many young piglets in some litters had weak legs, which splayed out beneath the piglet. Close inspection indicated that the problem was most prominent in litters derived from Landrace pigs. The problem suddenly appeared in several of these litters, with 10–20% of the piglets affected. The affected piglets appeared to be the smaller ones in the litters (Fig. 13.1i). The most common sign was piglets in which the two back legs splayed out sideways and forwards, causing the piglet great difficulty in standing up on its hind legs. The affected piglets tended to sit down and shuffle around on their back ends. This led to skin damage on the hind-quarters of these piglets. The farmer tied some tape around the back legs of these piglets to assist them to stand up (Fig. 5.13ii). In a few severely affected piglets, all four legs were weak and splayed out, so the piglet could not stand or sit and resembled a star shape. The pre-weaning mortality rate was increased, due to many piglets not being able to suckle properly and some were crushed by the sows.

Key Features

- Piglets in the first week of life with splayed legs.

5.13a. What is this problem?

5.13b. What control measures may assist the herd?

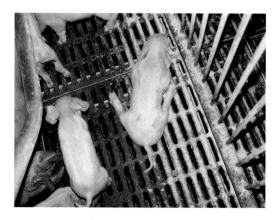

Fig. 5.13i. Smaller piglet with splayed hind legs.

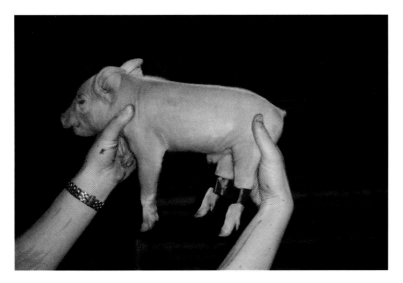

Fig. 5.13i. Piglet with splayed hind legs tied together.

5.13 Comments

5.13a. This condition is the common form of inherited leg weakness in piglets known as splay leg. The affected piglets suffer from a splaying out of the limbs soon after birth, which will severely limit their ability to move up to the teats and suckle, or to escape from under the sow. The specific causes of this problem are not clear, but it is more common in smaller, weaker piglets of the Landrace breed. These piglets appear to be born with a weakness in their adductor muscles in the pelvis area, which are the ones that keep the back legs together. This weakness is partly an inherited genetic condition, but may also involve various nutritional or other problems in the pregnant sow. It will be more apparent and damaging to piglets raised on wet and slippery floors.

5.13b. The survival of piglets with both the front and the hind legs affected is very poor and these piglets should be humanely euthanized. For piglets with only the hind legs affected, the hind legs can be tied loosely together above the ankle hocks with lightweight plastic tape. These piglets will often need assistance from farm workers to reach the teats and suckle colostrum in the first day of life. After suckling, these piglets can be removed and placed into a heated box area. After 1 or 2 days, these piglets with taped legs can then stand and hobble about and suckle milk alone. Massage of the hind leg muscles for 5 min every few hours, also assists the muscle recovery. If the piglet survives 5 days, then the tapes can be removed, the hind legs gradually become stronger and recovery will occur. A wide variety of methods to tape the legs together may be suggested to bring the hips and hind legs together, without blocking the anus or vulva. Without these various nursing interventions by caring staff, then many affected piglets will die.

The condition is partly inherited therefore the matings and boar used for production of these piglets should be noted and avoided. The floors of the farrowing pens should have sufficient grip for small piglets to move around easily. This may involve the provision of rubber matting around the sow in litters with the problem.

PART 6
Diarrhoea in Pigs After Weaning

6.1   Case Study

The farmer operated an established breeder, nursery and finisher farm system, on various connected sites. The farmer had purchased breeder pigs from a number of other farms over the past 2 years. For some months, the farmer noticed an increasing number of cases of diarrhoea and poor condition of the finisher pigs. Close examination indicated that 10–20% of the grower and finisher pigs ranging from 12 to 20 weeks old were thin, with 'sucked-in' flanks and poor body condition. Many of these pigs had severe diarrhoea (Fig. 6.1i). The diarrhoea consisted of loose sloppy faeces with many piles of faeces containing dark spots of sloppy watery blood and also thick spots of grey–tan coloured mucus (Fig. 6.1ii). When the sloppy faeces was grasped with hands, the mucus was slimy and stuck tenaciously to the fingers. Some of the breeder pigs in the farm units had similar clinical signs, with poor body condition and diarrhoea. The sustained level of serious diarrhoea and poor weight gains and associated costs led the farmer to consider the economic future of the farm.

Key Features

- Outbreak of diarrhoea and poor condition in finisher pigs.
- Sloppy faeces with dark blood and thick tenacious mucus evident.

6.1a. What is this problem?
6.1b. What control measures may assist the herd?

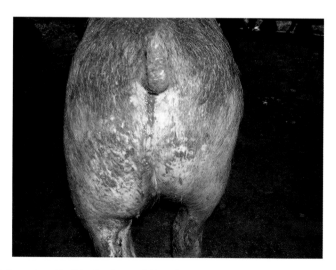

Fig. 6.1i. Finisher pig with thin flanks and bloody mucus diarrhoea.

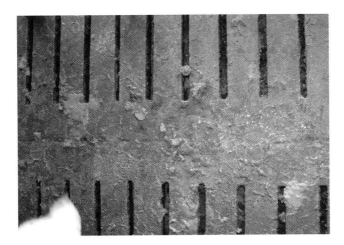

Fig. 6.1ii. Bloody faeces with thick mucus spots.

6.1 Comments

6.1a. This is muco-haemorrhagic colitis due to the snake-like spirochaete bacterium called *Brachyspira hyodysenteriae* (and closely related variants), and the disease condition is known as swine dysentery (SD). The somewhat older age groups affected and the clinical signs of rapid weight loss and bloody mucus-laden diarrhoea are distinctive. Post-mortem examinations will show that the distinctive muco-haemorrhagic lesions are confined to the large bowel. So the ileum and the stomach are normal.

The overall incidence of this infection in the pig industry worldwide declined greatly in many areas over the past 20 years, with the establishment of clean SD-negative breeding pig lines. However, the disease is making a strong comeback, because of movements of pigs from positive to negative production zones, changes in the organism itself, but mainly because of the regulatory-driven removal of most drugs that have been effective against the organism. The high economic cost of SD is associated with the marked depression of growth and feed conversion efficiency. Farmers may consider severe SD levels on the farm to be incompatible with sustaining the farm operation.

6.1b. Treatment for acute cases of SD must be provided via injections with tiamulin and followed up with use of tiamulin in the water and in the feed medication programme at 100 ppm. Alternatives to tiamulin are dimetridazole and carbadox, which are very effective when used in the feed medication programme. Lincomycin used at high dosages by injection or in the feed can also reduce clinical signs. SD vaccines are currently not reliable and are not recommended. Prevention on farms with endemic SD consists of providing one or more of the useful antibiotics in the weaner stages to reduce or eliminate SD infection in pigs, before they reach the later grower phases. Because SD can stay on the farm in carrier pigs and in rodents, it is not possible to eradicate SD without major cleaning and disinfection and a rodent control programme. SD is a disease amenable to eradication by intensive medication combined with intensive farm hygiene and biosecurity measures.

6.2 Case Study

The farmer operated an established nursery and finisher pig farm system, with groups of modern buildings holding many pens of pigs. The farm received weaner pigs from local breeder farms with modern lines of pig breeds. The farmer noticed that for some months many batches of growing pigs often had poor growth and moderate diarrhoea. Close inspection indicated that 20–40% of the 10–14-week-old pigs in the affected pens had a mild-to-moderate, sloppy, grey–green diarrhoea (Fig. 6.2i). No blood or mucus was evident in the diarrhoea. The pigs appeared relatively normal and active and appeared interested in food, but did not eat fully. There was noticeable variation among the weights of batches of pigs getting to the target slaughter-age weights, with many light-weight pigs left at the end of the fattening period. At autopsy of some of the more severely affected pigs, the farmer and veterinarian carefully examined the intestines and distinctive lesions were noted, consisting of thickening and proliferation of the internal lining mucosa of the terminal end of the small intestines (Fig. 6.2ii). The lymph nodes around these intestines appeared normal.

Key Features

- Variation in growth and sloppy loose faeces in growing pigs.
- Thickened mucosa of the ileum of affected pigs at autopsy.

6.2a. What is this problem?
6.2b. What control measures may assist the herd?

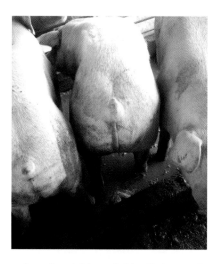

Fig. 6.2i. Groups of grower pigs of variable weight with loose diarrhoea.

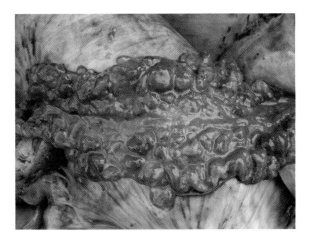

Fig. 6.2ii. Thickening of the mucosa of intestines of affected pig.

6.2 Comments

6.2a. The finding of moderate diarrhoea in grower pigs and thickened mucosa in the small intestine at autopsy is typical of proliferative enteropathy, also known as ileitis. This is a common bacterial disease of pigs worldwide caused by infection with *Lawsonia intracellularis*. The disease occurs commonly in all pig farm management systems. Infection of piglets probably occurs soon after weaning, via exposure to positive faeces. The infection can then amplify over the next few weeks in the groups of nursery pigs. It is likely that the environment of many pig farms contains a sustained level of *Lawsonia* infection embedded in faecal material sustained on farm equipment such as farm boots, the floors of pens, insects, rodents and walkways in the buildings; therefore transmission of positive faeces around farm systems can occur easily. This acts to consistently reintroduce the infection to each new batch of pigs, being more likely with frequent mixing and moving of pigs. Confirmation of the timing of infection can be performed by ileitis blood or PCR tests. Experience has shown that serology can be useful, in relation to the timing of possible interventions such as medication or vaccination. The incidence of ileitis lesions in pigs from affected farms at normal slaughter age is generally low, at 1–2% and therefore this technique is unreliable for farm monitoring.

6.2b. Treatment of ileitis is via antibiotics, particularly in-feed tiamulin or tylosin. The efficacy of these antibiotics is greatly enhanced when combined with strong pen and building hygiene and disinfection programmes. Use of antibiotic therapy to control the spread of clinical ileitis in weaner pigs during the post-weaning phase can be beneficial.

The ileitis vaccine (Enterisol ileitis®, Boehringer Ingelheim) has been shown to provide full immune protection to ileitis in grower and breeder pigs. Like all vaccines, the key to its successful usage is to provide plenty of time for immunity to develop after vaccination, but before infection. On many farms, it would need to be administered to pigs at around 2–3 weeks old. This vaccine can provide useful responses in terms of feed conversion and weight gains in the groups of growing pigs to slaughter age.

6.3   Case Study

The farmer operated an established breeding, nursery and finisher farm system on a single site, with a variety of older-style buildings and some outdoor pens. The farmer occasionally purchased breeder and weaner pigs from various local pig markets and small breeding farms. The farmers used all the pens regularly and pigs were moved around through different stages of the pig farms, with minimal cleaning or hygiene programmes. The farmer used various medication and vaccination programmes. The farmer had various older feed and grain storage areas around the farm, with many birds and rodents evident. The farmer noticed that over the past 6 months, an increasing number of groups of pigs around the farm were performing poorly and had diarrhoea (Fig. 6.3i). Close inspection indicated that in the nursery and finisher areas, 10–40% of the grower pigs in various indoor and outdoor pens had diarrhoea, were not eating properly and were in poor condition. The cases of diarrhoea were intermittent, with some pens having severe problems for a few weeks then some recovery, then reoccurring. The levels of mortality in these groups of pigs had noticeably increased. The type of diarrhoea was quite variable. In some pigs, the diarrhoea was somewhat watery and yellow, but in some other pigs, the diarrhoea was mucoid, sloppy and very smelly. At autopsy of some severely affected pigs, the lymph nodes around the intestines (mesenteric lymph nodes) appeared enlarged and the pigs had inflammation and thickening of their large intestine or colon. Examination of the mucosal lining inside the colon of some pigs demonstrated areas of ulceration and yellow necrotic membranes (Fig. 6.3ii).

Key Features

- Farm with older-style dirty areas and poor hygiene.
- Intermittent outbreaks of diarrhoea and poor condition in weaners and grower pigs.

6.3a. What is this problem?
6.3b. What control measures may assist this herd?

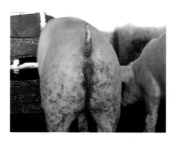

Fig. 6.3i. Pigs with sloppy diarrhoea in older-style farm buildings.

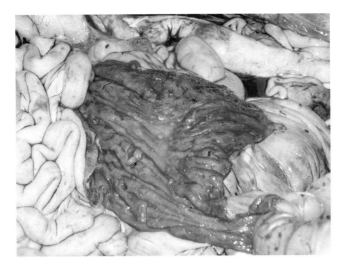

Fig. 6.3ii. Inflammation of large intestines with ulcers and necrotic areas.

6.3 Comments

6.3a. This is diarrhoea due to salmonellosis, with muco-haemorrhagic lesions in the large intestine. Salmonella are very tough bacteria and can survive in the environment of pig farms and in the intestines of many different animals for long periods. It is therefore a common infection of pigs and many other animals, such as rodents and birds. Many normal and healthy pigs are infected with Salmonella in their intestines during the grower and finisher stages, producing no diarrhoea or other specific health problems. Affected farms typically have had the infection for long periods and so have a history of salmonellosis. Clinical problems with diarrhoea in pigs due to salmonellosis are more likely in pig farms that have co-infections with one or more of the three immunosuppressive viruses that are common in pigs, namely PCV-2, PRRS or CSF. If the farm has poor hygiene programmes and uses outdoor pens or bedding for pens, then Salmonella levels in the pig pens can enable incoming pigs to receive a high dose at a young age.

Salmonella is easily isolated in a bacteriology laboratory from the intestines or faeces of affected pigs. In pigs, the usual bacteria involved are *Salmonella* Typhimurium and occasionally *Salmonella* Derby. Both of these are so-called Group B Salmonella. These bacteria are also easily isolated from the intestines of normal pigs at slaughter. Salmonella is therefore a potential food safety issue, if the intestines are ruptured and contaminate the meat portions of the carcass.

6.3b. Salmonella are difficult to control, and the infection persists on pig farms for long periods. Many Salmonella are resistant to some antibiotics, so the use of many different antibiotics on farms does not always reduce the infection in the herd. Salmonella vaccines have not been particularly useful for control of the infection or disease on pig farms. Also, the costs of vaccination on farms, may not translate to on-farm economic benefits. The most useful measure for control of Salmonella is therefore improvement of farm hygiene, with cleaning of manure pits, walkways and control of rodents and birds on the farm site.

6.4   Case Study

The farmer operated an established medium-sized breeder, nursery and finisher farm. There had been many different sources of pigs to the farm over the years, with various age groups and breeds now on the farm. The farmer had experienced a range of disease problems, therefore used a lot of pig treatments, but he was concerned about farm costs and did not use many commercial vaccines. The farmer noticed an increasing problem with poor condition and diarrhoea in some pigs through the finisher stages. Close inspection indicated that these pigs showed very poor growth rates, with some cases of diarrhoea. In most batches, the diarrhoea case problems seemed to be in grower and finisher pigs between 12 and 16 weeks old. The diarrhoea was usually yellow to green in colour, with no mucus or blood (Fig. 6.4i). At autopsy of pigs with diarrhoea, the pigs were in poor body condition, with thickening of the mucosal lining of the small and large intestine and greatly enlarged intestinal (mesenteric) lymph nodes (Fig. 6.4ii).

Key Features

- Cases of diarrhoea and poor condition in grower and finisher pigs.
- Thickened intestines and enlarged lymph nodes.

6.4a. What is this problem?
6.4b. What control measures may assist the herd?

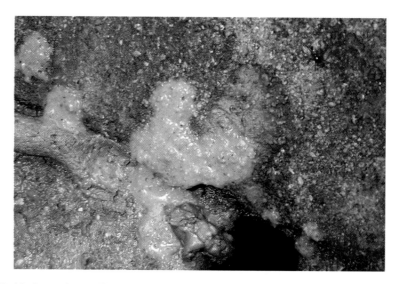

Fig. 6.4i. Moderate loose diarrhoea in some finisher pigs.

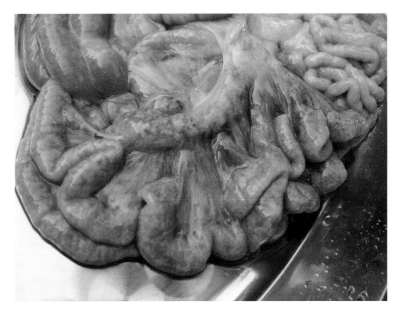

Fig. 6.4ii. Thickened intestines and enlarged mesenteric lymph nodes.

6.4 Comments

6.4a. This is wasting, diarrhoea and enlarged lymph nodes due to active infections with PCV-2. The thickening of the intestinal wall mucosa can be similar to that seen in proliferative enteropathy (ileitis), but the lymph nodes of pigs with PCV-2 disease are also always greatly enlarged. PCV-2 is a very common infection of pigs affecting farms all over the world. When this PCV-2 infection rises to a high level of virus in the blood and tissues, the damaging effects of the PCV-2 on lymph nodes and other tissues develop fully, with clinical signs occurring. The PCV-2 virus has several damaging effects on pigs. It has a direct damaging effect on lymph nodes, causing damage and necrosis and enlargement. This is connected with a strong immune-suppressive effect, causing a general reduction in the pig's ability to fight secondary infections. The recognition of the aetiological agent as PCV-2 and development of effective vaccines, has led to a dramatic reduction in the incidence of this wasting and diarrhoea problem.

6.4b. The affected pigs do not respond well to antibiotics or other treatments and should be culled. PCV-2 infection and its associated disease issues have been dramatically brought under control in pig populations in the past 10 years, by the introduction of effective commercial vaccines.

All farmers are urged to add PCV-2 vaccines to their vaccine list, as they are highly beneficial to the profitability of pig farming, when applied to the pigs in a proper manner. The sick pigs presented in this case study farm are therefore due to the farmer failing to use PCV-2 vaccines in a proper manner.

The main factors that cause PCV-2 infections to develop to a high level in some pigs are now considered to be the presence of co-infections (such as the common pig viruses, PRRS or parvovirus) and the pigs being of a susceptible breed, such as Landrace.

6.5   Case Study

The farmer operated a farm system consisting of breeding farms linked to nursery and finisher farm sites. The breeding farms had a successful programme of modern lines of pig breeds. The breeding pigs and the piglets received a full vaccination programme. The pigs were weaned at 3 weeks old and moved to the nursery areas. The feed mill decided to reduce the level of feed additives to the minimum levels, to save costs. Shortly after this, the nursery areas noticed serious problems with diarrhoea in batches of weaned pigs soon after they arrived from the breeding farms. Close inspection indicated numerous pigs in each new batch of weaner pigs had clear, watery, yellow diarrhoea (Fig. 6.5i). This diarrhoea started around 1–2 weeks after weaning. The diarrhoea shot out of the anus of these piglets, creating a projectile comet-like trail of diarrhoea. Some affected pigs remained reasonably alert and active, but others developed dehydration and shivering, and an increase in mortality levels was noted. The farmer and the veterinarian conducted autopsies of several weaner pigs with severe diarrhoea. They noted that many intestinal loops were dilated with watery, yellow fluid (Fig. 6.5ii), and that the local lymph nodes and the wall of the stomach appeared reddened and congested with blood. The skin of the pigs was blotchy and reddened in some areas.

Key Features

- The specific age range affected is 7–14 days after weaning.
- Yellow, watery, projectile diarrhoea.

6.5a. What is this problem?
6.5b. What control measures may assist the herd?

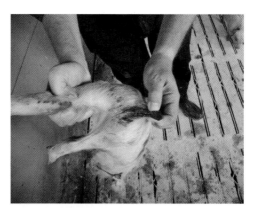

Fig. 6.5i. Watery, yellow diarrhoea in 5-week-old weaner pigs.

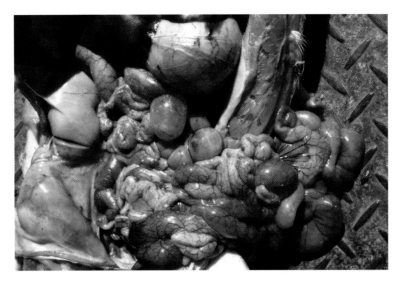

Fig. 6.5ii. Autopsy of affected nursery pig, with dilated loops of small intestine.

6.5 Comments

6.5a. The clinical signs and autopsy suggest that an ETEC had colonized many pigs' intestines shortly after weaning, causing cellular disturbances and watery, yellow diarrhoea. The *E. coli* vaccines used among breeder pigs are aimed for lactogenic immunity against ETEC in neonatal piglets and do not protect against ETEC infections in post-weaned pigs. So once the weaned pigs stop consuming milk and maternal antibodies, they quickly become susceptible to infections of ETEC acquired from the farm environment. Laboratory results can confirm bacterial cultures of lactose-fermenting, indole-positive, oxidase-negative and beta-haemolytic colonies of Gram negative *E. coli* from fresh intestine samples. The specific toxins and adhesins of ETEC are confirmed by agglutination reactions.

6.5b. Pigs affected with ETEC diarrhoea may be treated with suitable antibiotics, given by oral gavage or in-water therapy. Colistin is regarded as the drug of choice for ETEC therapy of affected groups of weaner pigs, with no clear indication yet of resistance among most isolates. Pigs may also be given rehydration fluids to assist their recovery.

E. coli and the ETEC strains are a common background organism that is considered to be 'embedded' in most pig farms, presumably in faecal materials in the pens, walkways and slurry. This embedded nature explains its constant nature of occurrence and outbreaks when appropriate control measures are not taken. The occurrence of clinical ETEC infections in post-weaned pigs had dropped away to a very low level since the 1980s with the introduction of in-feed zinc oxide at sufficient pharmaceutical levels (1500–3000 ppm) in early starter diets. Zinc oxide has a specific antibacterial action, damaging and distorting bacterial membranes with leakage of bacterial contents. However, some government initiatives aimed at environmental cleanliness have now led to limits in its general use, and an increase in cases of ETEC diarrhoea.

6.6   Case Study

The farmer operated a high-health status breeder farm, with modern lines of pig breeds. The breeding farm performed boar and gilt selection and developed young breeding gilts for multiplication of the breeding herd and sales to other farms. The health status of the breeder farm was excellent, with few major diseases. The farmer attempted to raise the breeding pigs with minimal use of antibiotics in the feed. The boars and gilts received commercial vaccinations against *Escherichia coli* and parvovirus. The farmer noticed occasional cases of dark, bloody diarrhoea, which had a rapid onset among groups of gilts or boars (Fig. 6.6i). The farmers who purchased gilts from the case study farm, also complained of similar cases of dark, bloody diarrhoea, which occurred in groups of gilts around 2 weeks after they arrived. Close inspection indicated that all these pigs had a dark, black–red, tarry and bloody discharge from the rectum. The affected pigs quickly became pale, with white eyelids, and many of these cases died. At autopsy of these pigs, the intestines were enlarged with marked thickening of the mucosa and serosal oedema (Fig. 6.6ii). The lumen of the ileum and colon often contained some large blood clots, but with no other bloody fluids or feed contents evident. The rectum contained black, tarry faeces. The mucosal surface of the affected portion of intestine showed little major damage, except for the marked thickening. No mucus, or bleeding points, ulcers or erosions were observed.

Key Features

- Dark, black–red, tarry diarrhoea.
- Mucosal thickening and blood clots in the ileum and colon.

6.6a. What is this problem?
6.6b. What control measures may assist the herd?

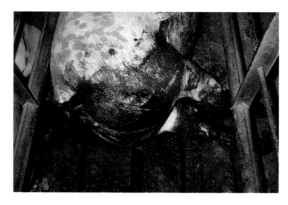

Fig. 6.6i. Dark, tar-coloured diarrhoea in breeder pigs.

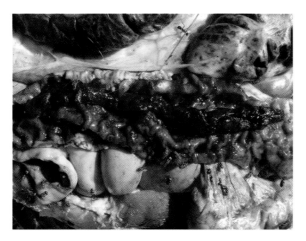

Fig. 6.6ii. Autopsy of affected pig, with thickened mucosa of intestine and blood clots.

6.6 Comments

6.6a. This is the acute haemorrhagic variant of proliferative enteropathy, also known as proliferative haemorrhagic enteropathy (PHE). As with the more common chronic form of proliferative enteropathy (ileitis), this disease is also caused by the intracellular bacterium, *Lawsonia intracellularis*. Cases of acute PHE occur most commonly in young adults at 4–12 months old, such as breeding gilts. These cases are marked by acute haemorrhagic anaemia with severe bleeding into the lumen of the intestine, but with typical underlying lesions of thickening of the intestine due to *Lawsonia*. The reason why some pigs develop this acute lesion has not yet been determined fully. Studies tracking *Lawsonia* infection on breeding farms have indicated that infected gilts or sows do not readily transmit the infection to their progeny in the farrowing area. The progeny from these affected breeding females are not protected from acquiring new cases of ileitis as growing pigs.

Particular management situations lead to reoccurring outbreaks of acute PHE, such as: (i) young adult pigs in boar- and gilt-performance testing stations; (ii) gilts within breeding programmes that involved transportation to new units; and (iii) the movement and mixing of boars and gilts into breeding groups. These serious outbreaks have become noticeably less common following the widespread usage of the live attenuated *Lawsonia* vaccine for breeding pigs.

6.6b. Treatment of PHE is via antibiotics, particularly injectable and in-water tiamulin or tylosin. The efficacy of these antibiotics is greatly enhanced when combined with strong hygiene and disinfection programmes. The *Lawsonia* vaccine (Enterisol ileitis®, Boehringer Ingelheim) has been shown to provide full immune protection to PHE in breeder pigs. Like all vaccines, the key to its successful usage is to provide plenty of time for immunity to develop after vaccination, but before infection. On many breeder farms, it would need to be administered to pigs at around 2–3 weeks old, with a booster dose at 6 months old. This attenuated vaccine is particularly important for introduction of replacement breeding stock into new premises. Previous use of acclimation and medication programmes in this situation led to many failures resulting in costly PHE outbreaks.

6.7 Case Study

The farmer operated an established finisher-fattener farm system that raised groups of larger pigs from 50 to 120 kg bodyweight. The pigs were raised in a variety of outdoor and indoor pens. Some of the older pigs were held in small outdoor pens for later sale as replacement breeder boars or females (Fig. 6.7i). Some of these pens had been used for this same purpose for several years. In some of these smaller outdoor pens with groups of around 20 pigs, the farmer noticed two or three pigs with diarrhoea. Close inspection indicated that the diarrhoea consisted of defaecation of large volumes of soft faeces, with visible amounts of blood and mucus in some of these droppings. The pigs in these pens were a mixture of weights, and some of the pigs appeared to be thin and slow growing. At autopsy of the affected pigs, they were in poor body condition with dark, bloody and mucus-filled colon and rectum. The colon of the pig appeared thickened and roughened. Close examination of the lumen surface of the colon when it was carefully washed, showed numerous small white nematode worms protruding from the mucosa (Fig. 6.7ii).

Key Features

- Small outdoor pens.
- Diarrhoea faeces with blood and mucus.
- Colon worms visible on close inspection.

6.7a. What is this problem?
6.7b. What control measures may assist this herd?

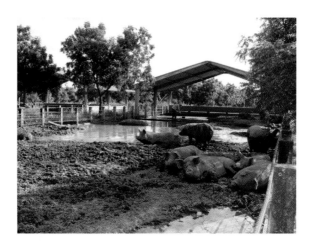

Fig. 6.7i. Pigs raised in smaller outdoor pens.

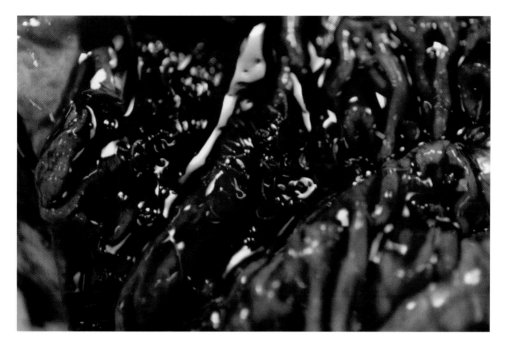

Fig. 6.7ii. Close-up picture of thickened colon with mucus and worms evident.

6.7 Comments

6.7a. This problem is the common whipworm of the pig colon, known as *Trichuris suis*. The variations in thickness of the worm segments give it the characteristic whip-like appearance. The life cycle of *T. suis* is direct and does not require any intermediate host in the environment. Whipworm eggs are passed in faeces from infected animals. These eggs are highly resistant and can remain viable in outdoor conditions for several years. Ingested eggs are taken in by the pigs and worm larvae penetrate and develop in the large intestine mucosa. The thin whip-like end remains embedded in the mucosal layers. The pre-patent period from ingestion of eggs until adult worms develop is 6–8 weeks. The disease is now mainly seen in smaller outdoor pens, with a high stocking rate. In this dirty situation, then the pigs may also have concurrent problems such as proliferative enteropathy (*Lawsonia intracellularis*), salmonellosis and other intestinal parasites including *Ascaris suum*. The clinical signs can closely resemble SD, which also causes a muco-haemorrhagic colitis, so great care must be taken to wash the colon and look for the visible portions of adult worms.

6.7b. Strategic rotation of outdoor pigs along with properly timed treatment with anthelminthics can reduce contamination of the outdoor pens. Whipworm eggs tend to stay in the upper 0–300 mm of soil, so this can be removed or covered by new soil, if space is limited. Clinical cases of trichuriasis in outdoor pigs appear to require a large infectious dose, so cases tend to be sporadic, unless pigs are kept for long periods in a small outdoor-pen area. Fenbendazole and ivermectin-type products are generally the most effective against *Trichuris* in pigs.

6.8 Case Study

The farmer operated a medium-sized breeder, nursery and finisher pig farm system on a single site. The breeder pigs on the farm were a long-established line derived from local breeds. The farmer maintained a good vaccination and medication programme for the pigs. The farmer also operated a feed-mixing and preparation facility on the same site (Fig. 6.8i), supplying all the different stages of feeds for the pigs. The farmer enjoyed negotiations with the local suppliers of all possible feed ingredients, such as cereals, fruits, soybeans, rice bran and various other by-products. Supplies of these items were stored at the farm and incorporated in various mixtures for each batch of feed. At one stage, the local price of soybean ingredients became much higher, and the farmer developed a batch of feed for grower pigs, containing only 10% cereals with significant amounts of beans and peas, as well as 20% of the diet consisting of canola extracts. Canola is also known as rapeseed plant. The grower pigs were fed this diet for several weeks. Nearly all of the pigs on this diet developed much softer, loose, sloppy, green faeces (Fig. 6.8ii). Close inspection indicated that all of the grower pigs in the group on this diet were affected with diarrhoea. Many of these pigs with diarrhoea grew slowly and some were in poor condition. Nursery and other finisher pigs on different diets did not have this diarrhoea problem.

Key Features

- Variable quality in pig diets.
- Sloppy, loose faeces in growing pigs on particular diets.

6.8a. What is this problem?
6.8b. What control measures may assist this herd?

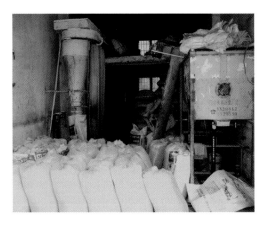

Fig. 6.8i. Farm feed-mixing facility.

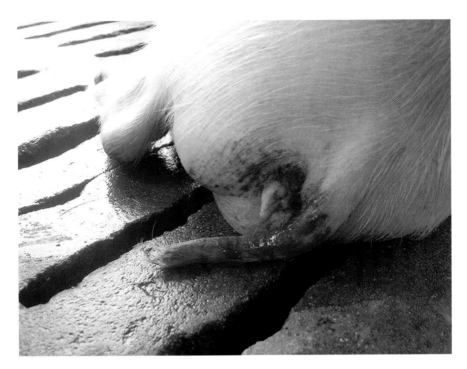

Fig. 6.8ii. Loose diarrhoea of many pigs in pens.

6.8 Comments

6.8a. The finding of moderate diarrhoea in grower pigs and poor choice of ingredients is suggestive of a nutritional imbalance leading to diarrhoea. Nutritional scours is generally a rare occurrence, but is often noticeable because nearly all pigs will be affected when given the particular batch of problem feed. Generally, a nutritional scour will be derived from a diet that has excessive amounts of indigestible vegetable protein. In modern farms this usually means excessive amounts of canola (rape) extract, or high protein soybean ingredients, or a variety of beans or peas of poor quality. Once the amount of indigestible protein in a pig diet rises above a level of around 15%, then the large intestine of the pig cannot process the diet fully and diarrhoea will occur. Some of these ingredients may also contain anti-nutritional factors. In a commercial feed-mill situation with full analysis of dietary ingredients, then these poorly digestible protein components should be kept at a low level.

6.8b. The incidence of nutritional scours will be reduced if pigs are fed a diet that has been fully formulated by a qualified nutritional expert, familiar with local and international sources of ingredients. Cereals and soybean ingredients and by-products are now the major components of pig diets around the world. If a farmer wishes to alter the types of cereals, protein and by-products sources to a more idiosyncratic formula, then they must be careful to keep the balance of the digestion of the pigs. The incidence of nutritional scours can also be reduced by use of modern, commercial genetic lines of pigs. These modern pigs tend to be more tolerant to higher levels of anti-nutritional factors.

6.9   Case Study

The farmer operated a medium-sized breeder, nursery and finisher farm system on a single site. The farmer occasionally purchased various sows and nursery pigs from other local farms. The feed for the pigs was derived from a variety of local sources. Groups of finisher pigs were sold to local markets, when they reached slaughter weight. The farmer had experienced a range of disease problems, therefore used a lot of pig treatments, but he was concerned about farm costs and did not use many commercial vaccines. The farmer noticed an increasing problem with poor condition and diarrhoea in pigs through the late nursery and early grower stages. Close inspection indicated that many of these pigs were dull and listless. Pigs seemed to slowly wander around in an aimless manner – the pig has nowhere to go and is in no hurry to get there. The pigs tended to lie down and huddle in piles. The pigs showed poor growth rates, with many cases of diarrhoea and several deaths (Fig. 6.9i). The problem seemed to mainly occur between 6 and 12 weeks old. The diarrhoea was usually loose to watery and of a dull yellow colour, with no mucus or blood. Some pigs also had sticky dark discharges noticeable at their eyes. Some sick pigs also appeared to have vomited yellow fluid. At autopsy of some of the pigs with diarrhoea, the pigs had empty stomachs and were in poor body condition, with some yellow fluids in their intestines. The kidneys seemed pale, with many small haemorrhages on the surface. The lymph nodes around the body also had some haemorrhages evident (Fig. 6.9ii). The problem persisted for some months, despite usage of antibiotics.

Key Features

- Dull nursery and grower pigs with yellow loose diarrhoea.
- Pigs with haemorrhages in lymph nodes and kidneys.

6.9a. What is this problem?
6.9b. What control measures may assist the herd?

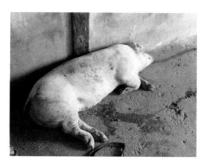

Fig. 6.9i. Depressed nursery and grower pigs with yellow diarrhoea.

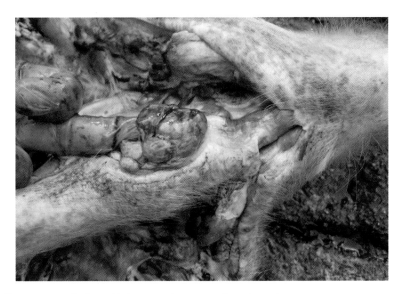

Fig. 6.9ii. Autopsy of pigs with haemorrhages on lymph nodes.

6.9 Comments

6.9a. This type of chronic diarrhoea and poor performing pigs is typical of the common form of CSF on a pig farm in an endemically infected region, where there may be many affected farms. In many herds, the breeding herd may be vaccinated with live attenuated vaccines or other local vaccines. In this situation, the piglets may have some immunity derived from the sow colostrum, but this immunity will fade after the pigs are 5 or 6 weeks old, then the nursery pigs will be infected and start to show these moderate clinical signs and diarrhoea. CSF infection will easily enter farms through contact with other pigs, contact with infected trucks or equipment. Pigs will also become infected if any infected pork product is somehow incorporated into their diet, perhaps by feeding of waste feed products to pigs. CSF can also be spread to groups of female pigs through use of infected boar semen.

6.9b. CSF is a very common disease in many parts of the world and can be difficult to control fully. Deaths and illness due to CSF will persist even if the farm uses a lot of antibiotics. A course of different CSF vaccines from international suppliers, such as the live attenuated C strain and the subunit E2 vaccines should be implemented. Full protection for CSF in endemic and high-risk pig farming areas, even with these vaccination programmes, is sometimes difficult. This is due to the fact that the disease is very common and pigs are exposed early in life, so vaccines may be administered at the same time as there is still some interference to protection, due to positive maternal antibodies. It is therefore often necessary to develop multiple vaccine points around the time of weaning and early grower period.

CSF is one of the three common viruses of pigs (along with PRRS and PCV-2) that cause immunosuppression of the immune system of pigs. A further problem is therefore that infection with PRRS or PCV-2 on a farm may also lead to a reduced efficacy of the CSF vaccines – and vice versa.

PART 7
Sneezing and Nasal Discharges in Pigs

7.1 Case Study

The farmer operated a medium-sized established farm on a single site, with various buildings for breeders, nursery and finisher pigs. The farmer often brought in extra breeder pigs and weaner pigs from nearby farms, to have periods of increased production. The farmer had a good medication and vaccination programme and good ventilation in the buildings. Following a long period of cool and cold weather, the farmer noticed that numerous nursery pigs around 4–7 weeks old were dull and had eye and nose discharges and were often sneezing (Fig. 7.1i). The problem seemed to start in one building and quickly spread to the other buildings. Close inspection indicated that 10–40% of the pigs in each building of the nursery herd were sneezing and had nasal and eye discharges. The nasal discharges were generally pale white with a mucoid to watery texture (Fig. 7.1ii). The affected pigs also had signs of lethargy, reduced appetite, with some coughing. The affected nursery pigs grew poorly but only a few died. At autopsy of these pigs, the farmer and his veterinarian noticed that the pigs also had mucoid exudate in their trachea and bronchial tubes, with scattered irregular areas of firm and dark purple consolidation in the front lung lobes.

Key Features

- Pig movements on to the farm.
- Pale mucoid nasal discharges and sneezing nursery pigs.

7.1a. What is this problem?
7.1b. What control measures may assist the herd?

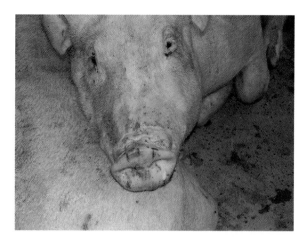

Fig. 7.1i. Sick pigs with nasal discharges and sneezing.

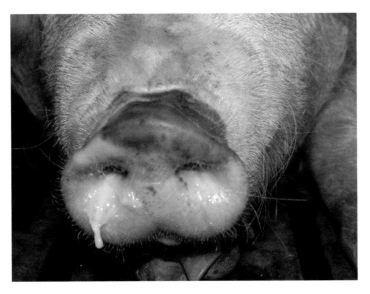

Fig. 7.1ii. Close up of pale white nasal discharge.

7.1 Comments

7.1a. This is an outbreak of sneezing, with nasal and eye discharges due to swine flu or orthomyxovirus influenza. This virus sets up a strong inflammatory reaction in the linings of the upper respiratory tract. The virus is then located and spread in the nasal secretions of infected pigs. It is a common infection among pigs all over the world. It is more common in regions with many pig farms and where pig movements occur between farms. This is because the swine flu virus does not form a long-standing infection and does not travel long distances. Swine flu therefore requires close and direct contact with pigs (snout to snout) to develop outbreaks, which are more common in the cold weather of autumn and winter. This form of swine flu is also commonly seen as part of a broader respiratory disease complex, with other infections such as PRRS.

7.1b. Groups of affected pigs may be placed into warm, well-ventilated areas and nursed until they recover. The use of antibiotics does not produce any specific response in affected pigs. A range of commercial swine flu vaccines are available for this disease. However, one problem is that swine flu is a disease where the milk of the sows will contain amounts of maternal antibodies, which will enter the blood of suckling piglets and block the action of any swine flu vaccine injection given to piglets. The swine flu vaccines are therefore usually more effective when they are given to breeder pigs rather than young piglets. A further problem is that there are various serotypes or variants of swine flu and these variants can change over time. The use of commercial vaccines must therefore match the same serotype that is present on the farms in the region.

The major factor to reduce outbreaks of swine flu is to reduce the numbers of times that pigs are moved and mixed with other pigs. One of the golden rules of pig farming is always – do not mix pigs.

7.2   Case Study

The farmer operated a medium-sized breeder farm system, which had several smaller breeder and nursery farm units on different sites. There was good farm biosecurity and an excellent medication and vaccination programme. The farm units had occasional cases of various pig health problems, such as virus infections and pneumonia. The farmer noticed some piglets between 2 and 5 weeks old were sneezing and had a nasal discharge (Fig. 7.2i). Close inspection indicated that several affected piglets had copious nasal discharge and strong violent sneezing. The nasal discharge was voluminous and varied from a sticky mucoid form to a more cheese-like, purulent form. These piglets had difficulty breathing easily and used their mouths to inhale air. Some pigs also had a watery eye discharge and some had swelling around the throat. Only a few of the affected piglets died during the period of sick and sneezing pigs. At autopsy of some of the badly affected piglets, the nasal cavity was opened with a saw and noted to be filled with the cheese-like pus and exudates (Fig. 7.2ii).

Key Features

- Piglets with mucoid and cheese-like nasal exudate.

7.2a. What is this problem?
7.2b. What control measures may assist the herd?

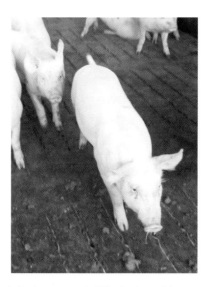

Fig. 7.2i. Piglets with nasal discharge and difficulty breathing.

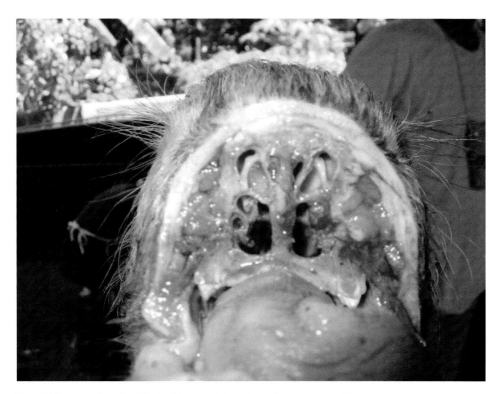

Fig. 7.2ii. Nasal cavity filled with mucoid and purulent cheese–like exudate.

7.2 Comments

7.2a. This is a viral infection of the nasal cavity (rhinitis) of pigs known as cyto-megalovirus or inclusion body rhinitis. It is a rare clinical problem, because any pig that is infected with this virus after the age of 3 weeks old will only develop an inapparent infection with a life-long immunity. So for a clinical problem to occur on a pig farm requires that this virus infection moves from one infected group to a group of naïve piglets, younger than 3 weeks old. So the clinical problems of cyto-megalovirus rhinitis, as described in the case study, will only arise sporadically on farms that may have been isolated or somehow become naïve to the virus. On some farms, piglets may be born with a more severe generalized form of the cytomegalo-virus infection.

7.2b. Some affected piglets may continue to show clinical signs and purulent rhinitis for several weeks, after the initial cases at 2–5 weeks old. There is no vaccine and no specific control measures. The clinical problem will usually dissipate, so no specific action is required in the face of cytomegalovirus infections.

7.3   Case Study

The farmer operated a large breeder and nursery farm system, in a region with many other pig farms nearby. The farm had a range of ongoing health problems, including swine fever and PRRS, which were partly controlled by vaccination programmes. The farm was located in a region that had numerous infections with foot-and-mouth disease (FMD) virus in pig farms and other livestock, such as neighbourhood cattle and goats. FMD was most common during the rainy season, when there were many movements of infected cattle. The farmer had previously had occasional outbreaks of FMD lesions on the feet of the pigs, but these were now controlled by a vaccination programme. The farmer noticed that during one rainy season, many of the breeder sows became lethargic and had a poor appetite. Many of these sows had mucoid nasal discharges and some were sneezing and had lesions on their snout (Fig. 7.3i). The affected sows lost condition and produced lower amounts of milk, but few deaths were noted. Close inspection indicated localized ulcerative lesions on the snouts of these older sows and finisher pigs (Fig. 7.3ii).

Key Features

- Pig farm in a region with a high level of FMD infections.
- Snout lesions on older pigs.

7.3a. What is this problem?
7.3b. What control measures may assist the herd?

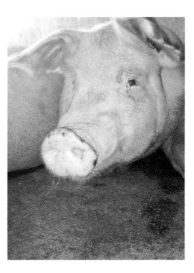

Fig. 7.3i. Older pig with snout lesions and nasal discharge.

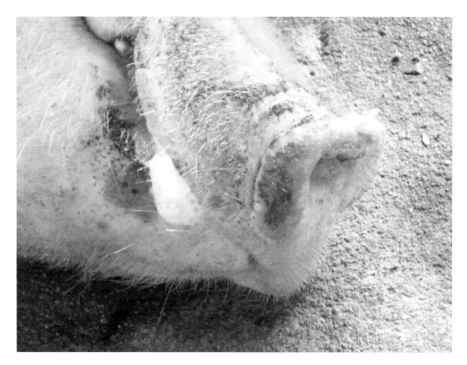

Fig. 7.3ii. Close up of snout lesions and nasal discharge in sow.

7.3 Comments

7.3a. These are moderate snout lesions and nasal irritation due to FMD in pigs. This syndrome, rather than severe foot or mouth lesions, is generally seen in sows or other animals that only have partial immunity. The sows may have some immunity from a vaccination programme for FMD. However, there is inevitably some variation in quality of FMD vaccines and vaccine storage and usage may not be optimal on all farms, leading to some sows with weaker immunity. Also, various strains or serotypes of FMD virus occur, which may lead to little or no cross-protection if the FMD vaccine strain is a different form of the virus.

Breeding sows will tend to have some innate resistance to FMD and may only show milder lesions, even in the face of a challenge from a high dose of FMD virus. High levels of FMD may circulate in regions with many infected farms, especially in certain seasons, such as rainy seasons when infected animals may move between regions. The infected pigs can amplify the virus and have huge amounts of virus in their expired breath. This can lead to FMD virus aerosols appearing over many pig farms and spreading to neighbourhood farms.

7.3b. FMD is highly contagious and is on the OIE list A of international trade. Any suspicion of FMD should lead to the farmer calling the government authorities, who may stop all movement of people and animals on and off the farm. Samples of lesions, other tissues and blood samples must be sent to designated laboratories in secure packaging for virus isolation and identification.

7.4 Case Study

The farmer operated an established medium-sized breeder, nursery and finisher farm, with various older buildings on a single site. The farmer had maintained a breeding and nursery programme with his pigs for many years, and often purchased replacement gilts and pregnant females from other smaller farms. The farmer used a minimal medication and vaccination programme. The farmer noticed that several groups of nursery pigs had sneezing and nasal discharges. Close inspection indicated that numerous pigs in some groups at 6–12 weeks old were snorting and sneezing. Many pigs had a serous to thick mucoid nasal discharge, and some pigs had bloody mixtures in this sneezing nasal discharge (Fig. 7.4i). There were also pigs with eye discharges, leading to dirty discoloured hair and skin below their eyes. Some of the pigs had some difficulty in closing their mouths properly. The pigs that had been affected for longer periods were growing slowly and some had noticeable deformities of their nose with a wrinkled nose or a twisted nose and snout (Fig. 7.4ii).

Key Features

- Nursery pigs with sneezing and mucoid-bloody nasal discharges.
- Nursery pigs with twisted nose and snout.

7.4a. What is this problem?
7.4b. What control measures may assist this herd?

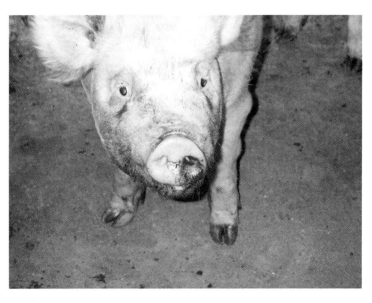

Fig. 7.4i. Pigs with sneezing and mucoid-bloody nasal discharges.

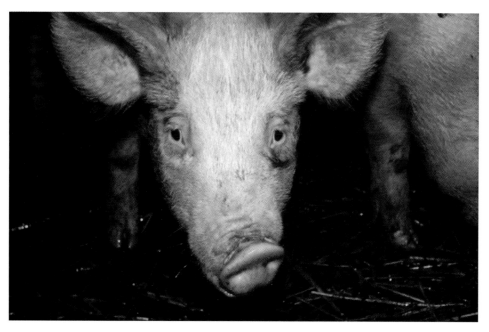

Fig. 7.4ii. Pig with twisted nose and snout.

7.4 Comments

7.4a. This is progressive atrophic rhinitis, which is a bacterial disease of pigs. It is unusual in that it is caused by a combination of two bacteria working together, *Pasteurella multocida* type D and *Bordetella bronchiseptica*. It is also unusual in that these bacteria have toxins that can specifically attack the bones and cartilage of the nasal turbinate bones. Most bacteria and viruses only attack soft tissues. The damage to the nasal bones leads to the highly distinctive twisting and wrinkling of the nose of affected pigs – enabling these pigs to sniff around corners. This disease was quite common on many farms up until the 1990s. However, this disease is now rare, for two reasons. First, there are many effective commercial vaccines that provide protection against the two causative bacteria. Secondly, there are now many lines and breeds of gilts and replacement pigs, which are free of the disease and are certified free. The disease is now mainly seen on older farms where piglets are derived from various sources of non-vaccinated gilts and are mixed together.

7.4b. The affected pigs may be treated with antibiotics, such as amoxicillin, that may control the two causative bacteria. In affected farms, the extent of damage to the nose may be examined in dead pigs at the slaughterhouse, by using a saw to cut across the upper face, at the level of the first premolar tooth. Use of commercial vaccines will usually control and prevent new outbreaks on farms that are positive. Restocking of the farm with pigs that are clean of the disease will lead to disappearance of the disease. The use of vaccines and restocking with these clean pigs means that a farm can become free of this disease and it seems to rarely return.

7.5 Case Study

The farmer operated an established nursery and finisher farm system, with groups of pigs housed in several older buildings (Fig. 7.5i). The ventilation and manure control systems on some of these buildings were becoming outdated and difficult to repair. Large groups of grower pigs were housed in the closed and dusty sheds in the colder winter months, on slatted floors, over deep manure pits and tanks that were now full of older slurry (Fig. 7.5ii). The farmer had not cleaned these manure pits or tanks for several years. The farmer noticed that many of these indoor pigs were sniffing and sneezing and had eye and nasal discharges. The hospital pens in these closed buildings had many pigs and the level of pig mortality in these buildings had increased during the winter months, with various cases of pneumonia and sick pigs. The farm workers also complained that these buildings were dusty and smelly and that if they stayed in the buildings for more than an hour, they also developed a nasal sniff and watery eyes.

Key Features

- Poorly ventilated and dusty, closed buildings.
- Nasal and eye discharges in pigs over full manure pits.

7.5a. What is this problem?
7.5b. What control measures may assist the herd?

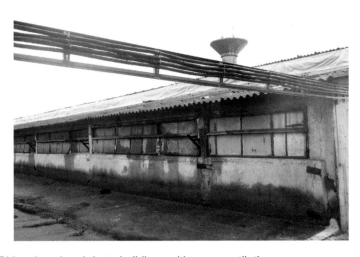

Fig. 7.5i. Older closed and dusty buildings with poor ventilation.

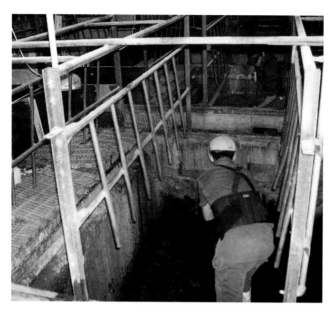

Fig. 7.5ii. Old sheds with workers in full manure pits.

7.5 Comments

7.5a. These are direct irritations of the upper respiratory tract caused by building dust and gases arising from manure pits in poorly ventilated buildings. The pigs in close contact with the dust and gases will suffer if the buildings are not properly ventilated to allow fresh air to enter on a regular basis. Besides the problems of excessive dust in closed pig farm buildings, there are two main gases that can arise from manure pits and irritate pigs and farm workers by direct irritation of nasal passages. The first gas is ammonia (NH_3). This is a common odorous gas found in pig environments, derived from decomposing slurry. At levels above 50 ppm inside a building, it irritates the mucosa of the eyes and nose. Repeated and prolonged exposure inside buildings will lead to sniffing and discharges in pigs and farm workers. The second gas is hydrogen sulfide (H_2S), which is also an odorous gas derived from decomposing slurry, particularly in tanks holding liquid manure. There may be a large release of toxic H_2S (rotten egg gas) whenever these tanks are agitated or removed. It is therefore vital to exclude any pigs and people from buildings and areas above these tanks, when these tanks are agitated or handled. Death can occur quickly in pigs or humans if the level of H_2S gas in the atmosphere goes above 200 ppm. A further gas that can occur in manure pits is methane (CH_4). This can reach high and foamy levels in deep manure pits if the feed of the pigs contains large amounts of dried distiller's grain extracts (DDGS). These soluble extracts are by-products derived from the fuel ethanol industry, which are placed into pig feeds. CH_4 is both an irritant and an explosive so the foamy CH_4 gas may catch fire or explode if an electrical spark occurs nearby.

7.5b. This is a farm management problem that is best addressed by attention to adequate safety procedures, farm maintenance and an ongoing building, manure-pit and ventilation-system replacement strategy. It is important to maintain proper ventilation and manure-pit operations, not only for the pigs but for farm-worker safety.

PART 8
Coughing in Pigs

8.1   Case Study

The farmer operated a medium-sized breeder, nursery and finisher unit in a traditional pig farming area, with many other farms in the region. The farmer maintained a stable breeder herd and raised the nursery and finisher pigs in various new and older buildings for the local markets. The farmer kept the pigs on a minimal medication and vaccination programme. The farmer noticed that over a period of 1 year, many of the grower pigs had developed a dry, persistent cough (Fig. 8.1i). The farm workers complained that it was very noisy to work next to these coughing pigs. Close inspection indicated that the coughing occurred in around 10% of pigs in most of the groups between 10 and 20 weeks old. The cough was a deep sound, and was chronic and non-productive. It seemed worse in pigs in the older buildings that had more dusty conditions. There was no major increase in mortality and the pigs were eating normally, but some pigs seemed slow at getting to slaughter weight. The farmer and his veterinarian inspected the lungs of batches of finisher pigs at the slaughterhouse and noticed well-demarcated, consolidated purple–red–grey areas in the front lobes (Fig. 8.1ii).

Key Features

- Groups of grower pigs with a deep chronic cough.
- Well-demarcated, firm, purple–red lesions in the front lobes of lungs.

8.1a. What is this problem?
8.1b. What control measures may assist the herd?

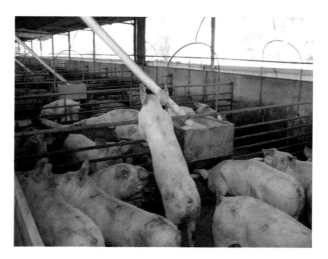

Fig. 8.1i. Groups of coughing grower pigs.

8.1 Comments

8.1a. This is enzootic pneumonia caused by the small bacterium *Mycoplasma hyopneumoniae*. It is the most common respiratory disease seen in pigs and is probably present in more than 80% of herds. The bacterium is easily spread a few kilometres by the wind between nearby farms or from pig trucks carrying live pigs. The disease is usually worse when pigs are kept in poorly ventilated older buildings. The diagnostic tests to confirm the presence of the bacterium, such as blood tests, PCR and culture, are not fully reliable in all situations. So the best practice is still to examine the lungs of pigs at the slaughterhouse, where it is possible to get a measure of the level of disease

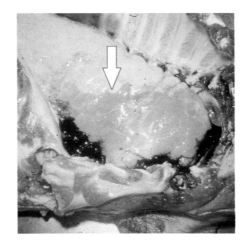

Fig. 8.1ii. Well-demarcated, firm lesions in the front lobes of the lungs.

on the farm. It is suggested to measure and compare the extent of damage in the lungs of 30–50 pigs. The lesions are seen as well-demarcated, solid, plum-coloured lung areas, fading to reddish grey as the lesions get older, with some mucus in the airways. These lesions are present in the front and ventral (lower) lobes. The remaining lungs may have some raised puffy pink areas. The case study illustrates a typical farm case, but occasionally, enzootic pneumonia may occur as a more severe outbreak, when the infection enters an isolated and naïve herd.

8.1b. Groups of affected pigs may be placed into warm, well-ventilated areas and treated with appropriate antibiotics, such as tylosin, tiamulin or lincomycin. It is also possible to place strategic medication into the feed or water for groups of pigs likely to be in danger of this disease, such as when pigs are mixed and grouped together. A range of *Mycoplasma* vaccines are widely available for this pneumonia disease. They are best given to pigs at 3–4 weeks old.

It is always important to have appropriate ventilation systems in pigs raised indoors, particularly where groups of growing pigs are raised together. Farmers must get appropriate advice on how to maintain and operate farm ventilation systems that bring fresh air to pigs on a constant basis. The development of all-in, all-out farm building systems, where groups of pigs do not mix, can also greatly reduce spread of the disease.

In some farms in isolated areas, it is possible to maintain freedom from this bacterium and disease. Pigs that are free of the bacterium may be purchased or delivered at birth, in a total depopulation–repopulation programme. Alternatively, the use of partial depopulation programmes involving hygiene and a strong antibiotic medication in the remaining pigs has also been shown to produce a successful eradication result. This eradication will lead to improved growth and performance of the growing pigs.

8.2 Case Study

The farmer operated a large farm system with breeder, nursery and finisher units on a single large-farm site. The farmer had purchased many gilts and developed various new lines of modern pig breeds. The nursery and finisher pigs were raised in various new and older buildings. The farmer noticed that over a period of 1 year, many of the groups of nursery and grower pigs were coughing. Close inspection indicated that the coughing started in around 10% of pigs in most of the groups between 6 and 12 weeks old. The cough was variable between pigs: some had severe persistent coughing that continued for weeks and others had a milder cough, with a gasping breath indicating the pigs had difficulty breathing properly. There was a moderately increased level of mortality in the batches of pigs. Occasionally, several pigs would die in a group in a 1 week period. Generally, the grower pigs seemed to be depressed with poor appetite and were slow at getting to slaughter weight (Fig. 8.2i). The farmer and his veterinarian inspected the lungs of batches of finisher pigs at the slaughterhouse and noticed various lung lesions. In some pigs, there was a diffuse firmness and a mottled, tan colour to all the lobes of the lungs, including the front and rear lobes (Fig. 8.2ii). In some pigs, there were also areas of fibrin and pleurisy over some areas of the front lobes.

Key Features

- Ongoing coughing and illness and deaths in grower pigs.
- Diffuse firm mottled tan-coloured lung lesions.

8.2a. What is this problem?
8.2b. What control measures may assist the herd?

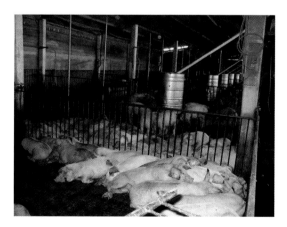

Fig. 8.2i. Groups of dull and coughing grower pigs.

8.2 Comments

8.2a. This is diffuse pneumonia caused by the PRRS virus. Since its emergence in the 1980s, this virus has become the number one health problem facing pigs around the world. The PRRS virus is a common infection in pigs around the world and has many strains. The PRRS virus is carried in the wind and is easily inhaled by pigs from the excretions of infected pigs. It is infectious even in small doses and from all secretions of pigs (saliva, faeces, aerosol, semen). There is commonly cross-transmission between different age groups, such as from breeder

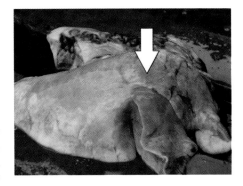

Fig. 8.2ii. Diffuse firm tan-coloured lung lesions.

pigs to nursery pigs. In nursery and grower pigs, it can cause a direct interstitial pneumonia, a type of pneumonia that attacks the blood vessels and linings of the airways in the lungs. The PRRS virus can also attack and harm the macrophages in the lungs. These cells are the ones that normally roam around the surfaces of the lungs grabbing and killing viruses and bacteria that enter the lungs, when the pig inhales air. So an outbreak of PRRS infections in a group of pigs can have many consequences for the respiratory system. This will include the diffuse pneumonia and also common secondary infections by other respiratory viruses and bacteria. All farms with PRRS infections in the lungs of their pigs will commonly have a range of respiratory diseases and raised mortality.

8.2b. The PRRS virus has proved difficult to control, particularly in areas where there are many pig farms in the region. Because there are many strains, and new strains are continually evolving, then having a recent outbreak of PRRS does not provide any immunity to the next PRRS virus entry and disease outbreak. It is therefore a common and ongoing problem.

It has proved possible to eradicate PRRS infections from breeding farms, by operating a completely closed herd and waiting for immunity to develop in the sows. After some months, these immune sows can then be inseminated with PRRS-negative semen and produce PRRS-negative litters of piglets. These piglets may be raised to become PRRS-negative nursery and grower pigs, if they are also kept fully isolated from other pigs. For a farm system to use this process requires good isolation of the farm sites and prevention of new infections in the future. It is therefore difficult to follow this programme in an area with many other pig farms nearby.

The control of PRRS therefore often relies on vaccines. Various PRRS vaccines are available. The modified live PRRS vaccines have been useful at providing some protection to pigs, which may be exposed to PRRS virus strains similar to the ones present in the vaccine. It is often important to establish what strain of PRRS virus is on the pig farm. This usually requires the use of PCR tests. For control of respiratory disease caused by PRRS, the vaccine may be applied to piglets at 3 weeks old. However, current vaccines do not prevent infections with all PRRS strains and disease can still occur in vaccinated pigs.

8.3   Case Study

The farmer operated a medium-sized nursery and finisher farm, with batches of weaner piglets entering the farm from different breeder farm sources. The farmer raised these nursery and growing pigs on a minimal vaccination programme. The farmer noticed that many of the nursery and grower pigs were growing slowly and that many had a gasping breath, with difficulty in breathing and some had a persistent cough (Fig. 8.3i). Close inspection indicated that these respiratory signs occurred in around 10% of pigs in most of the nursery groups between 7 and 12 weeks old. These affected pigs were generally dull and eating poorly. There was a noticeable increase in mortality through the nursery and grower phases. The farmer and his veterinarian inspected the lungs of affected pigs, at autopsy on the farm. The lungs of the affected pigs seemed firm throughout and had consolidated purple–red–grey areas in the front lobes, with some local pleurisy evident. The lymph nodes associated with the lungs, such as the nodes located in the midline between the two sides of the lungs, were greatly enlarged and firm and white (Fig. 8.3ii).

Key Features

- Groups of nursery and grower pigs.
- Ongoing coughing, poor growth and illness.

8.3a. What is this problem?
8.3b. What control measures may assist the herd?

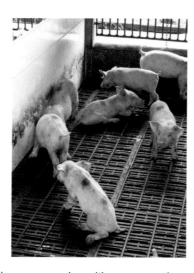

Fig. 8.3i. Groups of coughing nursery pigs with poor growth.

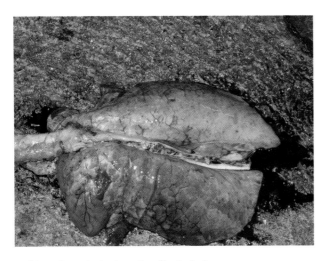

Fig. 8.3ii. Lung and lymph node lesions in affected pigs.

8.3 Comments

8.3a. This is pneumonia and lymph node damage due to PCV-2. This virus is a very common infection of pigs, affecting farms around the world. When this PCV-2 infection rises to a high level of virus in the blood and tissues, the damaging effects of PCV-2 on the lymph nodes and other tissues develop fully, with clinical signs occurring. PCV-2 has several damaging effects on pigs. It has a direct damaging effect on lymph nodes, causing damage, necrosis and enlargement. This is connected with a strong immune-suppressive effect, causing a general reduction in the pig's ability to fight secondary infections in the lungs. In nursery and grower pigs, it can also cause a chronic granulomatous pneumonia. Like the PRRS and the CSF viruses, this agent also acts to reduce the immune status of infected pigs. So an outbreak of PCV-2 infections in a group of nursery pigs can have many consequences, not only respiratory disease, but also more generalized diseases and wasting. So a farm with PCV-2 infections in the lungs of their pigs will commonly have a range of respiratory diseases and raised mortality. It is important to confirm the presence of PCV-2 in the lesions in the lungs and lymph nodes, usually by histology and PCR tests.

8.3b. The affected pigs do not respond well to antibiotics or other treatments and generally should be culled. PCV-2 infection and its associated disease issues have been dramatically brought under control in pig populations in the past 10 years, by the introduction of effective commercial vaccines. The most useful time for vaccination is around the time of weaning at 3 weeks old. All farmers are urged to add PCV-2 vaccines to their vaccine list, as they are highly beneficial to the profitability of pig farming, when applied to the pigs in a proper manner. The sick pigs presented in this case study farm are therefore due to the farmer failing to use PCV-2 vaccines in a proper manner.

The main factors that cause PCV-2 infections to develop to a high level in some pigs are now considered to be the presence of co-infections (such as the common pig viruses, PRRS or parvovirus) and the pigs being of a susceptible breed, such as Landrace.

8.4 Case Study

The farmer operated a medium-sized established farm on a single site, with various buildings for breeders, nursery and finisher pigs. The farmer often brought in extra breeder pigs and weaner pigs from nearby farms, to have periods of increased production. The farmer had a good medication and vaccination programme and good ventilation in the buildings. Following a long period of cool and cold weather, the farmer noticed that numerous pigs around 7–12 weeks old had an outbreak of coughing. The problem seemed to start in one building and quickly spread to the other buildings. Close inspection indicated that numerous pigs, 30–60% of the pigs in each building of the nursery and finisher herd, were coughing. Some pigs also had signs of lethargy, reduced appetite, with some eye and nasal discharges. The pigs put a lot of effort into their cough, with a deep hacking and paroxysmal cough effort and laboured breathing (Fig. 8.4i). Despite these dramatic signs, no finisher pigs died and many seemed to be recovering around 1 week after the start of the outbreak. When the farmer and veterinarian examined a few affected pigs at autopsy, these pigs had mucoid exudate in their trachea and bronchial tubes, with scattered areas of firm and dark purple consolidation in the front lung lobes (Fig. 8.4ii).

Key Features

- Pig movements on to the farm.
- Outbreak of deep hacking and paroxysmal coughing.

8.4a. What is this problem?
8.4b. What control measures may assist the herd?

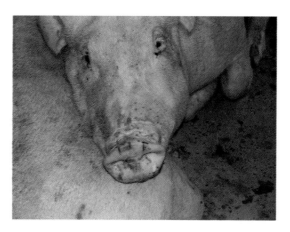

Fig. 8.4i. Numerous coughing pigs with a hacking and paroxysmal cough.

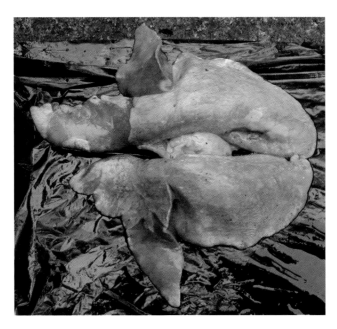

Fig. 8.4ii. Scattered areas of dark purple consolidation in lungs.

8.4 Comments

8.4a. This is an outbreak of coughing due to swine flu or orthomyxovirus influenza virus. This virus sets up a strong inflammatory reaction in the linings of the trachea and bronchial tubes. The virus is then located and spread in the nasal secretions of infected pigs. It is a common infection among pigs all over the world. It is more common in regions with many pig farms and where pig movements occur between farms. This is because the swine flu virus does not form a long-standing infection and does not travel long distances. Swine flu therefore requires close and direct contact with pigs (snout to snout) to develop outbreaks, which are more common in the cold weather of autumn and winter. The actual number of pigs affected in any outbreak can vary, from numerous pigs up to 90% of the herd, or in some other outbreaks, only a few pigs may develop the clinical coughing signs while the other infected pigs appear relatively normal.

8.4b. Groups of affected pigs may be placed into warm, well-ventilated areas and nursed until they recover. The use of antibiotics does not produce any specific response in affected pigs. A range of commercial swine flu vaccines are available for this disease. However, one problem is that swine flu is a disease where the milk of the sows will contain amounts of maternal antibodies, which will enter the blood of suckling piglets and block the action of any swine flu vaccine injection given to piglets. The swine flu vaccines are therefore usually more effective when they are given to breeder pigs rather than young piglets. A further problem is that there are various serotypes or variants of swine flu and these variants can change over time. The use of commercial vaccines must therefore match the same serotype that is present on the farms in the region.

The major factor to reduce outbreaks of swine flu is to reduce the numbers of times that pigs are moved and mixed with other pigs. One of the golden rules of pig farming is always – do not mix pigs.

8.5   Case Study

The farmer operated a large nursery, grower and finisher pig farm, which housed several hundreds of pigs in a variety of older buildings. The young nursery pigs arrived on to the farm in batches of transport trucks from one modern breeder farm. The main grower production pig growth was scheduled to take place from 10 weeks old until the pigs were 22 weeks old. The farmer occasionally used various types of antibiotics incorporated into the feed of these pigs. The farmer noticed that many of the older finisher pigs were coughing and had a poor growth rate (Fig. 8.5i). Close inspection indicated that many finisher pigs had developed a dry, harsh and persistent cough while in the grower pig period. These pigs seemed lethargic and did not move around easily, even when stirred by workers in the pens. The problem seemed worse in pigs raised in large groups in pens in the older buildings. The mortality level in the grower and finisher pig period was high, rising to 5% over the problem period. Many affected pigs had a slow growth rate and appeared gaunt. At autopsy of these dead pigs, the farmer and veterinarian noticed some dark black, haemorrhagic patches scattered in both the front and the rear lobes of the lungs (Fig. 8.5ii). There was some discoloration of these patches on the lungs, with a dark metallic sheen and pleurisy over these areas.

Key Features

- Deep, harsh coughing, exercise intolerance and increased mortality in finisher pigs.
- Dark haemorrhagic patches in the lung lobes.

8.5a. What is this problem?
8.5b. What control measures may assist the herd?

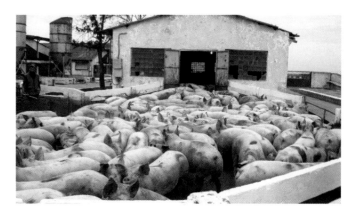

Fig. 8.5i. Groups of coughing finisher pigs.

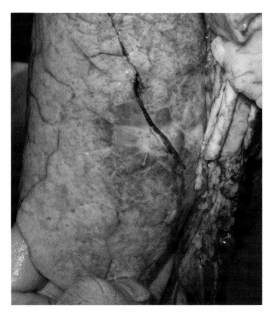

Fig. 8.5ii. Patchy haemorrhagic lesions in the rear lobes of the lungs.

8.5   Comments

8.5a. This is the more chronic form of pleuropneumonia caused by the bacterium *Actinobacillus pleuropneumoniae* (APP). Disease caused by APP is serious and common in pig farms around the world. The bacterium has many toxins which can have a strong debilitating effect on pig lungs. There are at least 15 known variants or serotypes of this APP bacterium. Many pig farms around the world are often infected with one of these serotypes, which are carried by sows in the breeder herd and transmitted to their piglet progeny. Some of these piglets will become fully infected and spread the disease quickly among the group. Some of the 15 APP serotypes are more serious and will cause a severe and deadly form of disease in grower and finisher pigs (see Case Study 3.8). However, several of these 15 APP serotypes will generally lead to the more chronic form of the disease in finisher pigs, illustrated in this case study. Also, the use of antibiotics among grower pigs that also have APP will reduce mortality and lead to this more chronic form of disease.

8.5b. Treatment of affected pigs is usually via use of injectable antibiotics, such as florfenicol, delivered to sick and coughing pigs. APP remains a common disease around the world affecting groups of finisher pigs. The APP bacterium is not easily removed from all pigs in groups by medications or vaccinations. APP has therefore not been reduced by the development of modern systems with purpose-built farm buildings, all-in, all-out batches and multiple site operations. The current commercial APP vaccines have not proved particularly useful at fully controlling the disease in all farm situations. Autogenous vaccines may be prepared from specific APP variants present on each farm, but this is a tedious procedure. Attention to improved ventilation of farm buildings and strategic use of antibiotics can help reduce the impact of the disease in most groups of pigs on an infected farm.

8.6   Case Study

The farmer operated a medium-sized breeder, nursery and finisher unit in a traditional pig farming area, with many other farms in the region. The farmer maintained a stable breeder herd and raised the nursery and finisher pigs in a few older buildings for the local markets. The farmer noticed that over the colder winter months, many of the grower and finisher pigs had developed a persistent cough and were growing slowly (Fig. 8.6i). Close inspection indicated that many pigs were dull and were moving around slowly for feeding. These pigs had a chronic, deep-sounding cough, and the pigs made a big effort to breathe normally, with some heaving of the chest in between periods of coughing. The coughing occurred in around 10% of pigs in most of the groups between 12 and 18 weeks old. The growth rates were slow and mortality levels had risen to 5% of the group in this period. It seemed worst in older buildings that had numerous groups of pigs in poorly ventilated and poorly heated conditions. The farmer and veterinarian inspected the lungs of batches of the affected finisher pigs at the slaughterhouse and noticed well-demarcated, consolidated purple–red–grey areas in the front and middle lobes of the lungs (Fig. 8.6ii). There were some areas of pale yellow pus in occasional areas of these consolidated lobes. There was also some pleurisy and thickening of the surface of these areas of the lungs.

Key Features

- Persistent deep cough and breathing difficulties in grower pigs.
- Dark consolidated lesions in the front and middle lobes of lungs.

8.6a. What is this problem?
8.6b. What control measures may assist the herd?

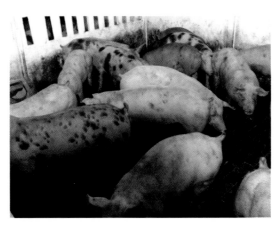

Fig. 8.6i. Groups of coughing grower pigs.

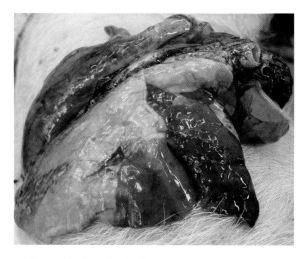

Fig. 8.6ii. Dark consolidated lesions in the front and middle lobes of lungs.

8.6 Comments

8.6a. This is advanced enzootic pneumonia caused by a combination of the small bacterium *Mycoplasma hyopneumoniae* with the common secondary bacterium, *Pasteurella multocida*. It is a common respiratory disease, especially seen in pigs raised in older and poorly ventilated buildings. *Mycoplasma* is a common infection and is probably present in more than 80% of herds. This bacterium acts to reduce the ability of the lungs to fight infections with other bacteria and viruses. Therefore coughing and respiratory disease situations in pigs often involve a mixture of infections, forming a complicated disease complex, rather than a single well-defined disease. The *P. multocida* bacterium involved in lung problems in pigs is usually the specific capsule strain A. These two bacteria (*Mycoplasma* and *Pasteurella*) are often resident on pig farms for many years. They may spread to new farms via pigs moved between farms. It is best practice to examine the lungs of pigs at the slaughterhouse, where it is possible to get a measure of the level of this common disease. It is suggested to measure and compare the extent of damage in the lungs of 30–50 pigs.

8.6b. Groups of affected pigs may be placed into warm, well-ventilated areas and treated with appropriate antibiotics, such as fluoroquinolones, tylosin, tiamulin or lincomycin. It is also possible to place strategic medication in the feed or water for groups of pigs likely to be in danger of this disease, such as when pigs are mixed and grouped together into the older buildings. A range of *Mycoplasma* pneumonia vaccines are widely available. They are best given to pigs at 3–4 weeks old. However, there are no effective vaccines for *P. multocida* type A.

It is always important to have appropriate ventilation systems in pigs raised indoors, particularly where groups of growing pigs are raised together. Farmers must get appropriate advice on how to maintain and operate farm ventilation systems that bring fresh air to pigs on a constant basis. If the disease occurs commonly in particular buildings, then the farmer must consider management responses to this health problem, based on construction of all-in, all-out pig flow in purpose-built farm building systems, where groups of production pigs do not mix. This will greatly reduce the spread and impact of the disease complex.

8.7   Case Study

The farmer operated a large farm system with breeder, nursery and finisher units on some adjacent farm sites. The farmer had developed various new lines of modern pig breeds and raised batches of nursery and finisher pigs in various new and older buildings. The farmer noticed that over the past 6 months, many of the groups of nursery and grower pigs had a higher rate of mortality. The death loss increased from 3% to 8% in the nursery and grower periods, with many coughing pigs. Close inspection indicated that the coughing started in 10–20% of pigs in some of the groups of nursery pigs between 8 and 12 weeks old (Fig. 8.7i). The cough was variable between pigs, but many pigs had severe persistent coughing that continued for many weeks, with gasping breath indicating the pigs had difficulty breathing properly. The coughing and mortality appeared worse in the batches of pigs raised in the older buildings. Generally, the grower pigs seemed to be depressed with poor appetite, several had a persistent cough and were slow at getting to slaughter weight. There was some reduction in the problems when antibiotics were given to the nursery pigs. The farmer and the veterinarian inspected the lungs of batches of finisher pigs at the slaughterhouse and noticed various lung lesions (Fig. 8.7ii). In some pigs, there was a diffuse firmness and a mottled, tan colour to all the lobes of the lungs, including the front and rear lobes. In some pigs, there were also areas of dark purple consolidation and fibrinous pleurisy with red–grey–purple areas of firm lung lobes and wide areas of fibrin and pleurisy and pericarditis. These lesions were scattered over some areas of the front, middle and rear lobes.

Key Features

- Groups of grower pigs in a pig-dense area.
- Ongoing coughing and illness.

8.7a. What is this problem?
8.7b. What control measures may assist the herd?

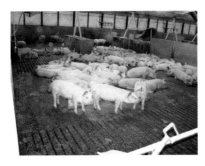

Fig. 8.7i. Groups of coughing and dull nursery pigs.

8.7 Comments

8.7a. This is PRDC, which often includes a combination of infections with the PRRS virus and strains of *Streptococcus suis*, which are adapted to the respiratory tract. This form of PRDC is common on pig farms around the world. The PRRS virus has a strong effect to reduce the immune function of pigs and so can 'open the door' to secondary pathogens that can cause the pneumonic pig seen on infected farms. Streptococci are common inhabitants of the throat of pigs,

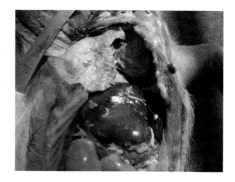

Fig. 8.7ii. Lung lesions in affected pigs.

and certain strains appear to be well adapted to enter the lungs of pigs and set up pathogenic infections. The combination of these two agents, and often others as well, is a common scenario for groups of pigs infected with PRRS. This can lead to a severe ongoing respiratory disease and health management problems. The PRRS virus is a common infection in pigs around the world and has many strains. The PRRS virus is carried in the wind and is easily inhaled by pigs from the excretions of infected pigs. It is infectious even in small doses and from all secretions of pigs (saliva, faeces, aerosol, semen). There is commonly cross-transmission between different age groups, such as from breeder pigs to nursery pigs. So an outbreak of PRRS infections in a group of pigs can have many consequences for the respiratory system. This will include the diffuse pneumonia and also common secondary infections by other respiratory viruses and bacteria. So a farm with PRRS infections in the lungs of their pigs will commonly have a range of respiratory diseases and raised mortality.

8.7b. The PRRS virus has proved difficult to control, particularly in areas where there are many pig farms in nearby areas. As there are many strains, and new strains are continually evolving, then having a recent outbreak of PRRS does not provide any immunity to the next PRRS virus entry and disease outbreak. It is therefore a common and ongoing problem.

The control of PRRS therefore often relies on vaccines. Various PRRS vaccines are available. The modified live PRRS vaccines have been useful at providing some protection to pigs, which may be exposed to PRRS virus strains similar to the ones present in the vaccine. It is often important to establish what strain of PRRS virus is on the pig farm. This usually requires the use of PCR tests. For control of respiratory disease due to PRRS, the vaccine may be applied to piglets at 3 weeks old. However, current vaccines do not prevent infections with all PRRS strains and disease can still occur in vaccinated pigs.

S. suis is a common infection on many pig farms around the world. There are no current vaccines that are effective for *S. suis*. Therefore strategic medication of weaner pigs is often needed to prevent damaging outbreaks. In-feed or in-water penicillin antibiotics are the most effective for this weaner medication programme.

The occurrence of streptococcal and PRRS forms of PRDC is often associated with mixing of weaner pigs from different sources. Therefore the development of farm management systems that streamline groups of weaner pigs from one breeder-farm source into a single nursery pig flow, with all-in, all-out management will generally reduce the number of cases of this common disease.

8.8   Case Study

The farmer operated a medium-sized nursery and finisher unit for pig production. The farm received weaner pigs from local breeder farms, with modern lines of pig breeds. The breeder pigs and young piglets all received a complete vaccination programme. The grower pigs were raised in groups of modern buildings, each housing several hundred pigs. The pig feeds were supplied in a high-density pelleted form by a large feed mill, with cereal, soybean and vitamin/mineral additive components. The feed mill used a fine particle-size mesh to prepare the high-density pellets, to ensure that the feed pellets did not crumble apart during transport and storage. The growing pigs were usually fed meals twice a day, at various times. The farmer noticed that a few of the larger grower pigs were coughing. Close inspection indicated that the pigs were generally healthy and eating, but the coughing in these few affected pigs was moderate and steady. The farmer and the veterinarian inspected the lungs of batches of these finisher pigs at the slaughterhouse and noticed small patches of consolidated purple–red–grey areas in the front lobes, with mucus in the airways and some focal areas of pus and fibrin tags in the affected lobes (Fig. 8.8i). On further inspection, there were also areas of moderate white thickening, roughening and erosions in the stomach of these pigs, at the oesophageal opening to the stomach (Fig. 8.8ii).

Key Features

- Moderate levels of OGU problems.
- Moderate levels of bronchopneumonia.

8.8a. What is this problem?
8.8b. What control measures may assist the herd?

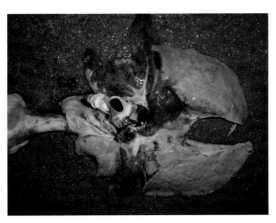

Fig. 8.8i. Moderate bronchopneumonia in the lungs.

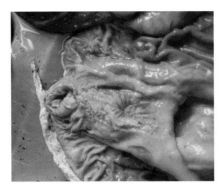

Fig. 8.8ii. Moderate roughening of the pars oesophagea of the pig stomach.

8.8 Comments

8.8a. These are cases of bronchopneumonia due to inhalation of gut bacteria into the lungs, which occurs during periods when the pigs are regurgitating food materials. This type of regurgitation is most common in groups of pigs that have mild or moderate lesions of OGU. The pig has a monogastric stomach. A rectangular-shaped zone in the stomach lining is known as the pars oesophagea, which surrounds the oesophageal opening. The glands of the stomach that secrete acid and protein enzyme (pepsin) are located in the main part of the stomach. This acid can rise up to attack the pars oesophagea, due to a combination of two main factors. The first factor is the type of modern feed produced at feed mills, which is often a pelleted high-density ration with a finely ground particle size, which improves the digestion and energy intake and the feed-handling characteristics. The second factor is a short cessation in feed intake (e.g. when the pigs cease feeding for a period of 1 day or more). This may be arise for many reasons such as: (i) hot weather; (ii) increased stocking density; (iii) feeder problems; (iv) the addition of some poorly palatable feed item; or (v) any disease problem.

In mild and moderate cases of OGU, there is only some thickening and irritation (hyperkeratosis) of the pars oesophagea. This causes reduced function of the junction between the stomach and the oesophagus, so bile and stomach materials will be regurgitated and can be inhaled, causing the bronchopneumonia cases. More severe forms of OGU are described in Part 3 (see Case Study 3.4).

8.8b. Pigs may be treated for OGU with the anti-stomach acid drug, ranitidine. This drug is widely available in various formulations, such as syrups, which may be given to pigs. Pigs with moderate bronchopneumonia may be treated with suitable antibiotics, such as florfenicol.

The control of OGU on a broader basis requires attention to feed quality, consistency and particle size. A larger particle size and increased roughage may be added to the feed mix. It is also important to pay attention to the various factors that may cause pigs to cease feed intake, even on an intermittent basis. This may be addressed by: (i) better temperature control for the pigs in hot weather; (ii) appropriate stocking density levels and sufficient feeder spaces; (iii) the removal of any poorly palatable feed item; and (iv) control of ongoing disease problems.

OGU remains a common problem on many larger pig farms, because pelleted feed is highly suitable for larger-scale operations and short cessations in feed intake can occur in groups of pigs, for many different reasons on most farms.

8.9 Case Study

The farmer operated an established outdoor pig farm, where groups of breeding and finisher pigs were raised on outdoor grass and soil-based pastures, which had some fence and pen divisions (Fig. 8.9i). The groups of pigs were moved around between different pastures at various intervals of 1–6 months. Each pasture had various feeder and watering stations for the pigs. The farmer purchased a group of new finisher pigs from a modern breeder company, to improve the lines of farm pigs, and placed them into one of the pig pastures. Around 2 weeks later, many of these newly introduced pigs became dull and developed a deep cough. Close inspection indicated that these pigs had a particularly deep, loud and harsh thumping cough, which the pigs continued in paroxysmal bursts. Some of the pigs also showed deep gasps involving their chest and abdominal breathing. The pigs did not recover and many lost body condition. The farmer and his veterinarian examined some of the lungs of these sick pigs at autopsy. The rear (diaphragmatic) lobes of the lungs had multiple focal dark lesions, with softer necrotic centres (Fig. 8.9ii).

Key Features

- Naïve pigs introduced to established outdoor pig pastures.
- Deep, harsh cough and lesions in the rear lobes of the lungs.

8.9a. What is this problem?
8.9b. What control measures may assist this herd?

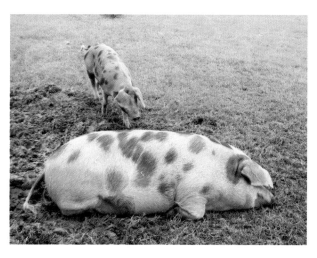

Fig. 8.9i. Pigs raised on fenced pastures.

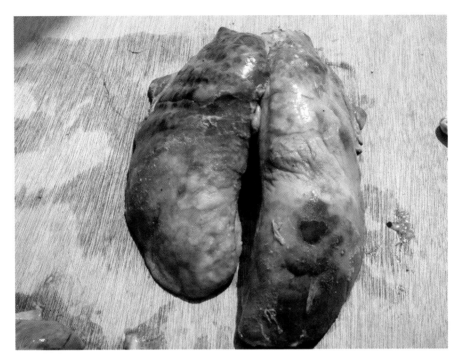

Fig. 8.9ii. Multiple focal necrotic lesions in rear lobes in lungs.

8.9 Comments

8.9a. This is parasitic pneumonia due to the damage caused by the larval forms of the common pig worm *Ascaris suum* migrating to the lungs. This worm occurs commonly in pigs kept outdoors or when pigs are raised on soil and bedding materials. The worm has a direct life cycle, wherein the worm lives in the pig intestines and its eggs sit on the pasture or bedding, waiting for the pigs to eat them. When the pig eats the worm eggs, they hatch into larvae which move around the pig's body on their way to the intestines. This worm is a large size and when the larvae of the worm move around the body, they cause direct damage as they chew their way through the liver and lungs. This particular form of coughing and pneumonia due to *Ascaris* is, however, quite rare, and requires large numbers of larvae to enter the lungs at the same time, to cause a noticeable and clinical damage to the pig's lungs. This will usually occur when naïve pigs are located on to a contaminated pasture and eat a lot of eggs at once, which then all hatch into larvae.

8.9b. The eggs of the *Ascaris* worm are practically indestructible on pastures, and can last many months and even years. Farmers operating outdoor pasture farms therefore need to pay attention to rotation of pens and pastures so that areas do not become highly contaminated. They also need to ensure that pigs are regularly given effective anthelminthic drugs, such as fenbendazole.

8.10   Case Study

The farmer operated an established outdoor farm system for finisher pigs, which were raised for sale and slaughter as larger pigs for retail ham production. The pigs were therefore raised in mixed groups of large fattening pigs up to 150 kg body-weight. The pigs moved around continually through various open pasture areas, and some orchard areas with old fruit trees and a few feeder and watering stations (Fig. 8.10i). The farmer noticed that several of the older fattening pigs developed poor body condition and a chronic, never-ending cough. Close inspection indicated that many pigs had slow growth rates, poor body condition, with a deep chronic cough and difficulty breathing. Antibiotic injections did not improve the cough or condition of the pigs. An autopsy was conducted on one of the worst-affected coughing pigs by the farmer and veterinarian. When the lungs and bronchial airway tree were opened, numerous 2–6 cm long thread-like worms were observed inside the airways (Fig. 8.10ii). The lungs had moderate pneumonia, with dark purple consolidation, which was particularly noticeable at the outer edges of several lobes.

Key Features

- Outdoor pigs with a deep hacking cough.
- Worms visible in the large airways of the lungs.

8.10a. What is this problem?
8.10b. What control measures may assist the herd?

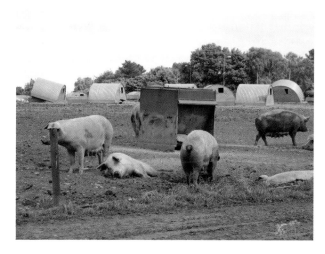

Fig. 8.10i. Finisher pigs raised on pasture areas.

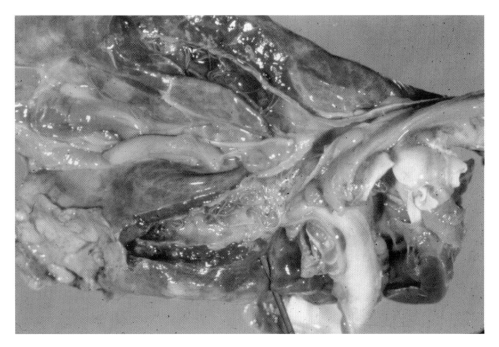

Fig. 8.10ii. Thread-like worms in the airways of the lungs.

8.10 Comments

8.10a. This is parasitic pneumonia caused by the specific lungworm of pig, named *Metastrongylus apri*. These worms live in the small airways (bronchi and bronchioles) of the pig lungs. These adult worms and their eggs and larvae produce an inflammation and irritant effect in the airways of the lungs, leading to the persistent cough. The life cycle of this worm is indirect, wherein the completion of the life cycle requires the intervention of earthworms on the ground. The life cycle is completed by pigs eating an earthworm that contains infective larvae inside it. Infection therefore only occurs where pigs have access to earthworms, for example in outdoor farms with open ground or orchards. While this may sound unusual, the disease is still common in some areas where pigs are kept outdoors. This is because the earthworm populations will retain the worms for long periods and pigs moving around on moist outdoor pastures are attracted by earthworms and will dig around trying to find them and eat them.

8.10b. The control of pig lungworm is simply by preventing access to infected earthworms in open-range farms. The levels of these worms in pigs are also controlled by use of anthelminthic drugs, such as fenbendazole. These drugs may be given to pigs in various formulations, such as in feed or by injections. The popularity and low capital costs of open-range outdoor production in some regions and countries, means that the pig lungworm is not rare in these places.

PART 9
Lameness Problems in Pigs

9.1 Case Study

The farmer operated an established grower and finisher farm with various older sheds that housed pigs from 30 to 100 kg bodyweight. Various groups of pigs arrived in batches at the farm site. The farmer had several other jobs, and used a range of casual labour to assist feeding the pigs. Over a period of several days, the farmer noticed that the growing pigs in all the farm sheds had become dull and lame. Close inspection indicated that nearly all of the pigs showed variable degrees of lameness and were lying down most of the time. When the pigs were forced to rise, they squealed loudly, hobbled about a little and did not move around. The pigs found it difficult to get to the feeders, had a much lower feed intake than normal and were losing condition. Some of the pigs appeared to be slobbering with excess saliva. When some pigs were caught and examined, dark bloody and ulcerative lesions were seen on the feet (Fig. 9.1i). In particular, these lesions were noted on the sides of their feet, just above the hoof, and sometimes in between the claws (Fig. 9.1ii). These lesions were more clearly visible when the feet were washed.

Key Features

- Lameness in a high proportion of pigs.
- Lesions on the sides of pigs' feet.

9.1a. What is this problem?
9.1b. What control measures may assist the herd?

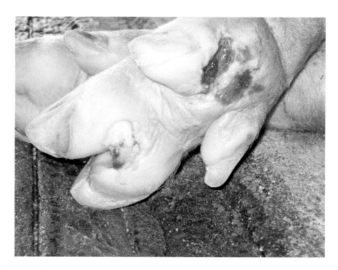

Fig. 9.1i. Dark and bloody ulcerative lesions on a pig's foot.

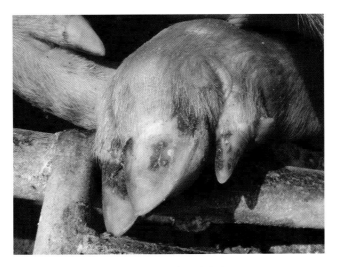

Fig. 9.1ii. Dark ulcerative lesions on the side of a pig's foot.

9.1 Comments

9.1a. This history and the clinical signs are suggestive of FMD arriving on to a pig farm site. FMD is characterized by a high fever and depression just prior to the onset of pronounced and severe lameness in groups of pigs. A highly noticeable feature of FMD in these situations is always the very high number of pigs affected in the group – it may approach 100%. The lameness is due to specific feet vesicle lesions, which appear as blanched, slightly raised areas on the edges of the hoofs. These expand and rupture in a short space of time, which leaves foot ulcers with shreds of torn tissue around the margin. These vesicle or blister lesions may also be seen on the snout, tongue and gums of some pigs. The lesions may also occur on the teats of sows in this stage, which will lead to cessation of suckling and deaths in the neonatal piglets. There are many serotypes of the FMD virus and even in endemic areas, on farms which may use vaccination, other new serotypes can arrive and cause this type of major new outbreak. Because of the rapid spread of this disease and its importance in international trade, it is important to get full information in all situations, such as:

1. What recent farmed animal movements on or off the farm have occurred?
2. Are other pigs on the farm affected?
3. Do any neighbouring farms have similar problems, which may include goats, cattle or sheep?

9.1b. FMD is highly contagious and is on the OIE list A of international trade. In any outbreak, many pigs are usually affected and they can provide a source of infection for other animals – pigs amplify the virus and have huge amounts of virus in their expired breath. This can lead to FMD virus aerosols appearing over pig farms and spreading to other farms in the neighbourhood. Any suspicion of FMD should lead to the farmer calling the government authorities, who may stop all movement of people and animals on and off the farm. Samples of vesicle fluid, other tissues and blood samples must be sent to designated laboratories in secure packaging for virus isolation and identification.

9.2   Case Study

The farmer operated an established and older-style breeder farm, with various modern lines of breeder sows. The farm buildings for the gilts and sows in the gestation and mating areas consisted of various old wooden-sided sheds and some outside pens next to these sheds. The floors in these areas were a mixture of solid concrete and some wooden structures. Some of these floors had poor drainage areas and some had also become rough and worn over the years of use. In previous years, the farmer had noted that the annual rate of culling and mortality among the sow numbers was around 5%. However, in the current year, the farmer noticed that once or twice a month, one or more pigs would become lame, with a swollen foot. The overall annual mortality rate in the sows had currently risen above 10%. Close inspection indicated that affected pigs were usually large, heavy pigs kept in the older dirty pens and initially had a reluctance to put weight on one of the hind feet. Over a week or so, the affected foot was noticeably larger and hot and painful and the sow did not rise (Fig. 9.2i). The swollen foot and hoof eventually formed abscesses and bloody ulcers just above the hoof (Fig. 9.2ii). The sow remained lame, did not eat properly and was usually culled.

Key Features

- Dirty pens.
- Lameness in larger pigs with enlarged ulcerated toe.

9.2a. What is this problem?
9.2b. What control measures may assist these pigs and the herd?

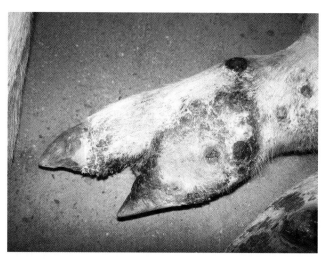

Fig. 9.2i. Enlarged hind foot of a heavy sow kept in an older pen.

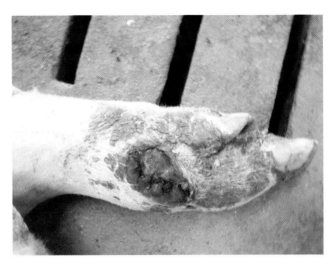

Fig. 9.2ii. Enlarged hind foot with ulcerated abscess.

9.2 Comments

9.2a. This is suggestive of an abscess inside the foot of the pig – a condition that is also known as septic laminitis. This is a common problem in some farms, and it usually arises where larger pigs may stand their hoof in dirty areas of manure in pens. If there is any crack or opening in a toe in the foot, then this leads to contamination of the inner part of the toe hoof with bacteria from the environment. These are not specific bacteria, but a range of *Escherichia coli* and many others present in manure and environmental materials. Once they enter, these bacteria will then grow inside the hoof and form an abscess, which will swell and burst just above and around the hoof. The condition is more likely where the floors or slats are old and rough, as this will abrade and damage the toes, and so open up cracks and openings. It is also more likely when floors in the breeding or farrowing areas are wet and slippery and the sows may hurt their soft hoof when they attempt to rise. Also, pigs that are too fat, or with deformed feet, will put excess pressure on the hoof and create openings. In addition the diet of modern sows should contain appropriate nutrients for proper hoof growth. If these nutrients are at a too low level the hoof can be more susceptible to damage.

9.2b. When affected pigs are identified, the affected hoof and toe can be made dry and clean and the pig given a strong course of injectable antibiotics. The antibiotics, such as lincomycin, can be given in high doses for at least 5 days. The pigs can also be given painkillers, to assist them in moving around and enabling them to eat properly. The foot abscess may be opened up by surgical methods, but these types of abscess in pigs are often fairly dry and so this surgery generally does not assist the individual pig. The experience is often that once a foot abscess develops, it is difficult to cure and the lesion may become worse, even with treatment.

For prevention, the sows should be kept active and in good condition in clean, dry and well-drained pens, without any rough areas that may abrade the feet. The diets of all pigs should contain adequate biotin and zinc for proper and tough hoof growth. Suggested levels would be at least 300 µg biotin/kg of feed and 100 mg soluble zinc/kg of feed in the sow diets throughout the year.

9.3   Case Study

The farmer operated a modern breeder farm system, which was expanding the numbers of the breeding gilts with new lines of clean female gilt pigs. One of the gilt multiplier farms was in an isolated region, with excellent modern buildings, biosecurity and nutrition. The farmer noticed that in some groups of these gilts, at around 15–25 weeks of age, many pigs in the group showed varying degrees of lameness (Fig. 9.3i). Close inspection showed that around 10–20% of the pigs lay down frequently, were reluctant to stand and some had difficulty in rising up (Fig. 9.3ii). This lameness seemed to mainly affect the larger, well-muscled pigs. The pigs had no external lesions, swellings or sores on their feet or elsewhere. The affected pigs were losing condition, compared with their condition when they arrived. These pigs seemed to have difficulty moving easily to the feeders, due to their lameness. However, they mostly seemed to recover after 2 weeks of clinical signs. The problems seemed to be worse in colder weather periods.

Key Features

- Modern breeder farm system.
- Pigs reluctant to stand with some loss of condition.
- Moderate numbers of affected pigs within groups at 3–6 months old.

9.3a. What is this problem?
9.3b. What control measures may assist the herd?

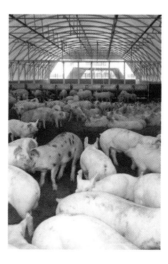

Fig. 9.3i. Groups of larger pigs at 15–20 weeks old.

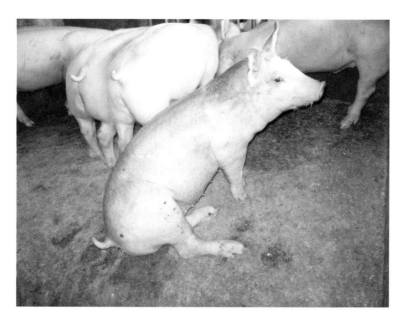

Fig. 9.3ii. Pig reluctant to stand and bear weight on its legs.

9.3 Comments

9.3a. This is inflammation of the joints (arthritis) caused by the small bacterium *Mycoplasma hyosynoviae*. The feature of lameness in many pigs in a group at 3–6 months old is characteristic. It is likely that the agent is present in most herds throughout the world, but it only seems to cause clinical signs in a minority of herds, particularly groups of gilts. It is generally a fairly mild disease resulting in lameness and consequent reduced feed intake for a period of 2 weeks or more in the affected gilts. Deaths are rare, and many animals recover fully with or without treatment. However, it can be costly, as the farmer cannot sell or use some of these lame gilts at this important time for breeding programmes. The arthritis is more severe in heavily muscled pigs, who are also likely to get other leg problems, such as osteochrondrosis, a non-infectious degenerative disease of the joints.

The disease seems to be more common in modern farm systems, with some segregated breeder farm production. This type of system may lead to more pigs that are not exposed to the organism earlier in life, and so there is no immunity in the gilts. On smaller traditional or older-style farms with all ages of animals present together in one site, pigs become naturally infected at a young age, by contact with the organism in nasal secretions from older animals. These pigs will then develop a strong immunity and so the disease is not common in these traditional farm systems.

9.3b. This *Mycoplasma* is a small bacterium that causes joint inflammation and pain. The bacterium is sensitive to several antibiotics, such as lincomycin or tiamulin, but it is not sensitive to penicillin. Treatments are best given by individual injections to the pigs, and injectable anti-inflammatory products may also be given to help the lame pigs move around and eat. *M. hyosynoviae* is a separate and different agent from *Mycoplasma hyopneumoniae* which causes enzootic pneumonia. The *Mycoplasma* that causes arthritis is therefore not controlled by the *Mycoplasma* pneumonia vaccines.

9.4 Case Study

The farmer operated an established breeding, nursery and finisher farm system, with a range of older buildings for the pigs. The farrowing pens were poorly maintained, with the floors and pen walls becoming worn. The farrowing areas were busy and the staff generally only had time to perform a minimum level of duties inside the farrowing rooms and pens during the day. The farm manager was inexperienced and used many untrained labour staff for piglet processing – that is cleaning, castration, injections and teeth-clipping procedures after farrowing (Fig. 9.4i). The farmer noticed that the pre-weaning mortality was becoming high, with an increase of 1–2% extra mortality above the background level of 13%. The main cause of losses appeared to be an increase in lame piglets with swollen joints. Close inspection indicated that some younger piglets less than 1 week old were reluctant to stand up and held up a leg when they walked. These piglets could not reach the sow teats easily and lost condition and some were cases of overlay by the sow. In piglets that were 2 weeks old and older, several were noticed with an enlarged swelling of the main joints, such as the knee or ankle (Fig. 9.4ii). These swollen joints persisted in the older piglets, and they moved around slowly, with a loss of body condition. If the swelling burst, then some dry yellow pus came out from the affected joints. Some affected piglets also had swellings around the navel area.

Key Features

- Older-style farrowing area and inadequate care taken when processing piglets.
- Lameness and swollen joints in piglets.

9.4a. What is this problem?
9.4b. What control measures may assist the herd?

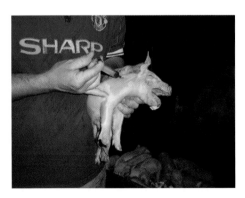

Fig. 9.4i. Piglet processing by untrained staff.

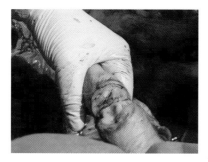

Fig. 9.4ii. Swollen and thickened leg joint in a young pig.

9.4 Comments

9.4a. The key features are suggestive of joint ill, which is an inflammation of the joints (arthritis) affecting one or more joints, usually in young piglets. The cause of the infection in the joints is usually common environmental bacteria such as *Escherichia coli*, staphylococci or streptococci. These bacteria will initially enter the bloodstream then settle down as an infection in the larger joints. These bacteria grow and form a reaction consisting of a pus-filled joint. There are various ways that environmental bacteria can gain initial access to the bloodstream of young piglets. The farrowing area may be poorly cleaned and not hygienic. The piglets may have dirty navel areas if they are not cleaned properly soon after birth. The piglets may develop wounds and abrasions on their feet from old and rough floors. The various procedures in the processing of piglets in the first few days of their life also provides opportunity for these bacteria to enter via wounds at the navel or teeth-clipping, tail-docking or castration sites. Joint ill at low levels is a common problem on many farms. However, an increase to a point where it is noticeable and affecting farm performance, suggests that the care and processing of piglets is not fully adequate or hygienic.

9.4b. Individual affected piglets may be given appropriate injections of antibiotics such as penicillin for 3–5 days. Some piglets do not respond to treatment and should be culled.

Attention to farm hygiene is the critical control measure. In terms of piglet processing, then some control measures would include dipping of the navel in iodine shortly after birth. This may require attention by both night time and day-time staff in farrowing areas. The floors of the farrowing areas should be clean and dry. Cleaning procedures of the farrowing pens need to be reviewed and adequate disinfection and drying times allowed. Some farms also use dry mats and disinfectants in the farrowing areas, but these may not be a complete cleaning material. Farms should regularly repair or replace any worn floors, especially old concrete or slats. The use of sharp and clean specialized scalpel or clipping instruments, antiseptic hygiene, wound dressing and staff training is vital for all piglet-processing procedures such as teeth clipping, tail docking and castration. These procedures should be done at 1–5 days of age, but not before 6 h of age. The use of a dosage of antibiotics for all piglets at this time is also performed on some farms, particularly where joint ill is a problem. However, this may lead to the development of antibiotic resistance among some bacteria on the farms.

9.5 Case Study

The farmer operated a large breeder and nursery farm system, with modern farm buildings. The breeding pigs were from modern hybrid breed lines and had few problems. The farrowing rates and average numbers of piglets born alive and numbers of pigs weaned were at a good level. The pigs were weaned at 3 weeks old and mixed into groups raised in large nursery sheds. The farmer noticed an emerging problem in pigs in these nursery units, with outbreaks of lameness in pigs at 5–8 weeks old (Fig. 9.5i). In one typical group of 1500 weaner pigs, 20% were counted as being lame. Many of these pigs had swollen knee and ankle joints, which were painful for the pigs. The pigs appeared dull and feverish. Several of these pigs became more unwell and died. When these pigs were examined and some of these joints were opened, there was a large amount of cloudy cream-like pus in some joints and some yellow, watery fluids in other joints (Fig. 9.5ii). Some of the pigs seemed to respond to injections of penicillin.

Key Features

- Lameness and swollen joints in young weaner pigs.

9.5a. What is this problem?
9.5b. What control measures may assist the herd?

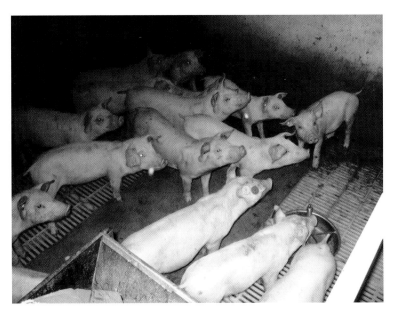

Fig. 9.5i. Groups of lame weaner pigs.

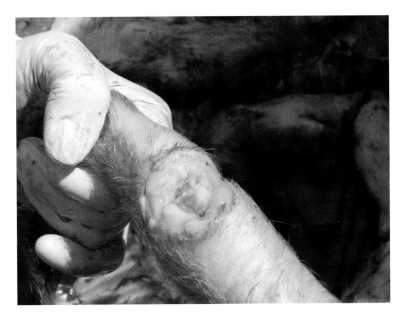

Fig. 9.5ii. Swollen and fluid-filled joints.

9.5 Comments

9.5a. These signs are suggestive of post-weaning joint inflammation caused by the common bacterium *Streptococcus suis*. This is a common problem on many farms, but it is often sporadic with outbreaks that can disappear and then reappear. Streptococci bacteria live in the environment of many pig farms in the dust and faecal materials in sheds, as well as in infections among healthy carrier pigs. This may include infections of the vagina of many sows. Therefore, many farm pigs become infected with *S. suis* in the bloodstream as young piglets and when they are mixed in new groups at weaning. This new infection can occur via the throat tonsils and the pigs may not have appropriate immunity levels. After the bacterium enters the bloodstream, it can settle into one or more of the larger joints, usually in young weaner pigs. Some particular strains of *S. suis* appear to be more likely to go to the joints, and start an inflammation with a pus reaction and swelling. This bacterium is easy to culture and identify in routine laboratory situations from samples of fresh pus materials from an affected pig joint – provided it has not been treated with antibiotics.

9.5b. Individual pigs that are affected with streptococcal arthritis may be treated with injections of long-acting penicillin. If the pig is treated early in the course of the disease, then a recovery rate of around 50% may be expected. There are no effective vaccines for *S. suis*. The most useful control programme for prevention of the disease is addition of penicillin-type antibiotics into the feed of pigs in the period after weaning. The occurrence of the disease is usually made worse when pigs from many different breeding farms or areas are all mixed together at weaning. This creates a situation where many different strains of *S. suis* mix around in a group of pigs. It is therefore an important aim of nursery and weaner pig management to fill sheds with streams of pigs from a single source.

9.6   Case Study

The farmer operated a large modern breeding farm, with clean and modern buildings. The farm had an active breeding programme of modern breeds of pigs, with matings and lines of pigs with an emphasis on rapid growth, lean muscle percentage and meat flavour. This breeding aim led to a rise in the numbers of Duroc and Landrace breed pigs, so these pigs were now the majority of the breeding herd. Over the past 6 months, the farmer noticed that the rate of culling of breeding males and females was increasing. The main reason noted for the culling was chronic lameness, particularly among the Duroc pigs, for both males and females (Fig. 9.6i). The problem seemed worse when pigs were moved across longer distances between different areas of the farm, such as sows returning from the farrowing areas back to the mating areas. Close inspection of these affected pigs indicated that they often walked in short steps, with the front part of their body in a swaying motion and other abnormal gaits. The more severely affected pigs were seen to lie down a lot, on their side or squat down on their front legs, and have difficulty rising up (Fig. 9.6ii). The pigs did not respond to injections of antibiotics or anti-inflammatory drugs. At autopsy on some affected pigs, the farmer and veterinarian noticed excess joint fluids and a bilateral and symmetrical lesion of erosions in the joint cartilage and growth line (epiphysis) in the main bones in the elbows. Similar lesions were also seen on the cartilage of the medial femur condyles in the knee joints.

Key Features

- Modern breeder farm system.
- Moderate numbers of affected pigs at 4–6 months old.
- Signs of leg lameness and loss of condition.

9.6a. What is this problem?
9.6b. What control measures may assist the herd?

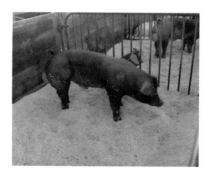

Fig. 9.6i. A heavy-muscled Duroc pig.

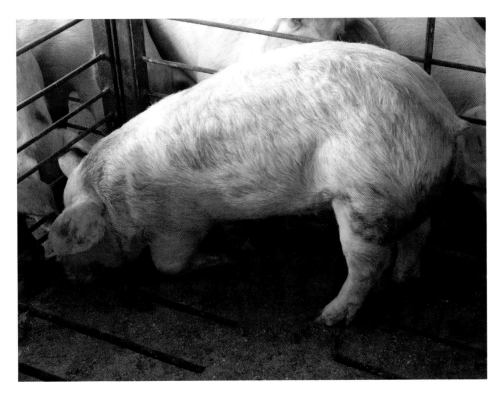

Fig. 9.6ii. A heavy-muscled pig that is lame in the front-leg elbow joints.

9.6 Comments

9.6a. This type of lameness is caused by osteochondrosis dissecans in pigs. This is not an infection, but it is a degenerative change that occurs in the cartilage and growth lines of the large bones of the pig body, particularly in the areas of the bones forming the elbow and knee joints. It is common in larger breeds, particularly in the Duroc and Landrace. It appears to be mainly an inherited problem that is passed down between the matings of specific lines of pigs in these breeds. It is less common in the Large White breed (also known as the Yorkshire). The genetic problem consists of a defect in the maturation of cartilage cells in the growth plates of these long bones around the main leg joints. It is made worse when large, heavy pigs, both males and females, are made to exercise by walking or during natural mating programmes.

9.6b. The breeding programmes of pig farms should take into account the overall survival rates of the pigs and look to reduce major causes of mortality or culling, such as these inherited forms of lameness. The diet of the pigs appears to have little influence on the problem. The addition of Large White pigs into the breeding programme may assist the reduction of this problem.

9.7   Case Study

The farmer operated a large breeder farm, which had been expanding over the past 10 years, with modern breeds of pigs. The farm had various older buildings and walkways that had been repaired over the years. Some of these walkways and pens had older concrete floors, with up- and down-slopes and bare, slippery patches. The farmer noticed that many of the gilts and sows in the breeding herd had moderate lameness, and were not eating well. Close inspection of these gilts and sows when they moved between the different areas of the farm indicated that they had a short stride, with uneven steps and stiff legs. These pigs also bobbed their head up and down and swayed their body when they walked. When standing, they held their back arched and shifted weight on their feet. Close inspection of the feet of these pigs showed that they had visible cracks in the horn walls of the claws. These cracks were present in mild to severe forms in around 20% of the gilts. The cracks commonly occurred in specific sites on the feet: (i) a vertical claw crack; (ii) a horizontal claw crack (often with some haemorrhage) (Fig. 9.7i); or (iii) around the softer ground-facing heel and sole of the feet (Fig. 9.7ii). In some sows, there was also some over-growth of one of the toes, or damage to the dewclaws.

Key Features

- Chronic lameness in developing gilts and sows.
- Cracks and similar lesions in the claws and sole of the feet.

9.7a. What is this problem?
9.7b. What control measures may assist the herd?

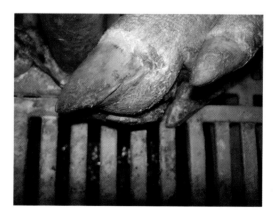

Fig. 9.7i. Typical crack in a claw.

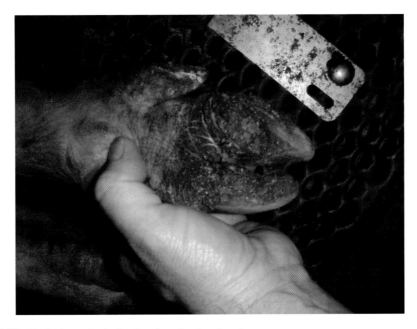

Fig. 9.7ii. Typical cracks in the heel and sole of a claw.

9.7 Comments

9.7a. These are cases of lameness due to feet problems in breeder pigs. They are common problems and seen on many breeder farms, particularly those with older concrete floors. Each foot of a pig consists of four digits or claws, of which only two (digit 3 and 4) contact the ground. The hoof comprises a hard wall and on the ground-facing side, a softer sole and heel. The visible junction of the hoof wall and the skin of the leg is known as the coronet. Cracks will develop in these structures if the feet of the gilt do not develop properly and the feet are stressed by movements around rough floors, and wet, slippery conditions. In some farms, keeping the pigs on soft, damp floors can have similar effects, with poor claw development and cracking. There is also some evidence that proper nutrition over the periods of growth of the legs, feet and claws of gilts is important for full development of a firm and tough claw hoof.

9.7b. The proper nutrition of gilts and sows plays an important role in prevention of lameness due to feet problems. The hoof wall is continually growing, so this nutrition needs to be ongoing. The key elements appear to be an appropriate amount of both biotin and zinc, as well as amino acids. The amino acids are the building blocks of the hoof proteins and the biotin and zinc are important trace elements needed in the hoof formation process. The amino acid levels in pig diets are supplied by the protein content from animal or plant sources, such as soybeans, often supplemented with synthetic amino acid mixtures. A minimum level of dietary biotin for sows raised on concrete is considered to be around 300 µg biotin/kg of feed and for soluble zinc around 100 mg zinc/kg of feed. The zinc for this requirement should be in a soluble form, such as zinc sulfate, not the insoluble zinc oxide form. In some herds with particular claw problems, it can be suggested to raise the biotin levels by double or triple this recommended amount.

9.8 Case Study

The farmer operated a large modern breeding farm, with clean and modern buildings. The farm had an active breeding programme of modern breeds of pigs, with matings and lines of pigs looking for an emphasis on fertility, rapid growth and lean muscle percentage. This breeding programme saw a big rise in the numbers of Landrace breed pigs, so these pigs were now the majority of the breeding herd. Over the past 6 months, the farmer noticed many cases of severe lameness, particularly among the Landrace pigs, for both males and females (Fig. 9.8i). The severe lameness problem seemed to occur exactly around the time of first matings involving these pigs. Close inspection of these affected pigs indicated that they had been slow and lame but then had suddenly developed a more severe hind-leg lameness problem. They often sat down on their back legs, and were seen to lie down a lot, and were highly reluctant to rise up. One side of the hip region of the pigs often seemed more painful to the touch. This painful leg seemed to be slightly shorter than the other hind leg. The pigs did not respond to injections of antibiotics or anti-inflammatory drugs. At the autopsy of an affected pig, the inside of the affected hip joint had marked haemorrhage and inflammation, with a fracture of the neck of the femur bone at this area of the hip joint (Fig. 9.8ii).

Key Features

- Modern breeder farm system, with occasional affected pigs at 4–6 months old.
- Acute and severe pain in hip joint of larger pigs.

9.8a. What is this problem?
9.8b. What control measures may assist the herd?

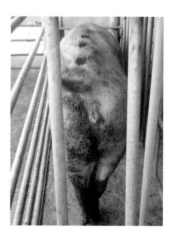

Fig. 9.8i. Sow with severe lameness in one hind leg.

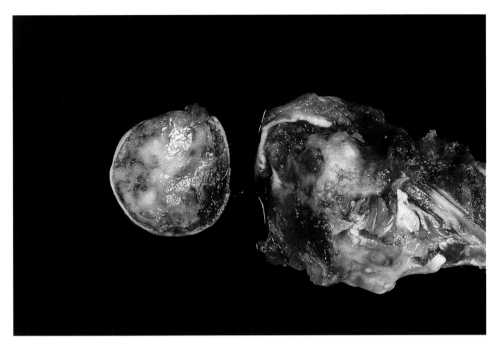

Fig. 9.8ii. Lesions in the hip joint – haemorrhage and damage to the neck of the femur.

9.8 Comments

9.8a. This is severe lameness due to damage to the top ball-shaped head of the femur leg bone, known as femoral head epiphysiolysis – a degeneration and breakage of the head of the femur in pigs. This is not an infection; rather it is a degenerative change that occurs in the cartilage and growth lines of the large ball-and-socket joint at the hip of the pig body. The cause of the disease is therefore similar to that of osteochondrosis dissecans, which occurs in other large bones and joints of pigs, such as the elbow and knees. This femoral-head problem is common in larger heavily muscled breeds, particularly in the Landrace and Duroc, and is less common in the Large White (Yorkshire) breed. It appears to be mainly an inherited problem that is passed down between the matings of specific lines of pigs in these breeds. The genetic problem consists of a defect in the maturation of cartilage cells in the growth plates of this leg bone around the main hip joint. It is made worse when large, heavy pigs, both males and females, are made to exercise by walking or during natural mating programmes. The acute form of this disease, demonstrated here in this case study, in some pigs is due to the head of the femur coming to a point where it detaches from the rest of the femur, creating a movable and highly painful loose attachment inside the hip joint. Usually, this femoral-head detachment only occurs on one side initially.

9.8b. The breeding programmes of pig farms should take into account the overall survival rates of the pigs and look to reduce major causes of mortality or culling, such as these inherited forms of lameness. The diet of the pigs appears to have little influence on the problem. The addition of Large White pigs into the breeding programme may assist the reduction of this problem.

9.9   Case Study

The farmer operated a large and established breeder farm, consisting of sows of different lines and breeds. The farmer had become more focused on the boar section of the business, so there was an increasing size and number of buildings housing an expanding number of young boars. The boars and the semen production were used for both the farm sows and in sales for other pig farms. Some young boars were housed in groups and others in individual boar pens. Some of the mating and mounting pens for the boars were newer pens, but many of the mating pens had been converted from old finisher pig pens. These converted pens were smaller, had slippery floors and still had their feed and water troughs (Fig. 9.9i). The farmer noticed that at least 20% of the younger boars did not perform male reproductive work, despite repeated efforts to guide these boars by several farm staff. These boars were consistently reluctant to mate and mount either the sows in the mating pens, or the dummy used for semen collection. The boars generally were eating well and had few other health problems. Close inspection indicated that these younger boars seemed to have slight lameness and various injuries and problems with their legs. These leg problems seemed to consist of a range of individual boar problems, such as lacerations or bite wounds on their flanks and legs, fracture or damage to a dewclaw, fracture in a toe, large cracks in a hoof (Fig. 9.9ii), or painful areas around some joints.

Key Features

* Younger boars in small mating pens.
* Boars slightly lame and reluctant to mount sows.

9.9a. What is this problem?
9.9b. What control measures may assist the herd?

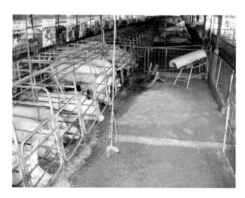

Fig. 9.9i. Mating area with slippery floors.

9.9 Comments

9.9a. The boars of some lines and breeds are considered more lazy and sluggish in reproductive work, than other breeds. It is suggested that around 10% of normal boars never become particularly adept at reproductive work in modern farm settings, and these boars may be culled. Boars work best when routine and consistent training and mating or mounting practices are maintained. This scenario of individual cases of lameness in young boar pigs, therefore usually relates to a series of

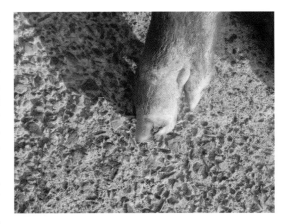

Fig. 9.9ii. Large crack in the hoof of a boar.

management issues in the raising, training and mating procedures for boars. It occurs most commonly when there are problems in training of boars and when there are design problems in the mating pens. These will include mating pens that have wet, slippery floors, and where farm tools and equipment, or the pen fixtures, such as feed and water troughs, increase the chance of collisions and impede simple mating progress. These design problems may also be sharp corners and areas in the mating pens, where the sows can hide and make natural mating more difficult. It will also occur where a smaller younger boar is placed into the mating pen with a large aggressive sow, who will attack the boar.

9.9b. The training of younger boars for reproductive work is important. Boars raised in same-sex groups will show aggressive and homosexual behaviours to each other. This will lead to injuries and poor condition among some of the boars. When boars and sows are placed in mixed-sex groups, it is important to compare the size of the boars and the sows, so that sows do not assume a dominant social position. The body size of the young boar must be adequate to cope with mounting of the dummy or mating of larger female pigs. The young boar must be fully acclimatized to the mating or mounting areas, before any reproductive work is commenced. It is important not to expect boars to perform reproductive work shortly after feeding. It is therefore recommended to feed boars after mating procedures or to wait 2 h after feeding, before reproductive work. This gives the boar time to partly digest his feed and perform toilet functions (but not sleep), prior to mating procedures. The reproductive work should be performed at cooler times of day. The farmer and his team have to spend long periods checking and watching these younger boars and actual mating procedures. Some boars will be deterred from subsequent matings if they are injured, fatigued or pushed around, by larger, aggressive or uncooperative sows.

In an ideal mating or mounting pen there are: (i) smooth corners; (ii) no fixtures or other objects to collide with; and (iii) firm, non-slip floors. Many farms use mats or bedding materials to improve the floors.

9.10 Case Study

The farmer operated a large modern breeder farm with various lines and breeds of modern pigs. Various lines of hybrid pigs were selected for entry into the breeding programmes at around 20 weeks old and later mated in breeding programmes. The reproductive performance of these pigs was normal, with good farrowing rates and numbers born alive. However, the culling rate in the selection process of some of the new lines of younger gilts was high. The reason for this high culling rate was mainly problems with poor gait and lameness in the gilts. Close inspection indicated that many of the new breeding gilts had problems with the conformation of their legs and spine, in comparison with normal gilts. Some affected gilts had a high arched back, rather than the flat top and level back that is desired in normal gilts. Other gilts had back legs that formed a straight-line position, with these pigs appearing to be on tip toes (Fig. 9.10i). Other gilts had low shoulder position problems, with the scapula positioned more directly over the front legs, leading to weak front legs (Fig. 9.10ii). Many of these gilts with poor conformation had narrow bodies and shorter bones in the lower legs, with more evidence of feet problems and hoof cracks, compared with normal.

Key Features

- Increased culling rate of gilts in modern breeding programme.
- Gilts with poor conformation of spine, hind legs and front legs, compared with normal.

9.10a. What is this problem?
9.10b. What control measures may assist this herd?

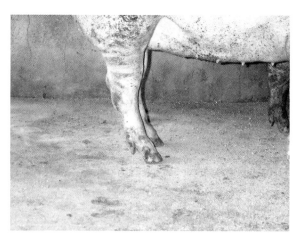

Fig. 9.10i. Gilt with poor conformation of back legs.

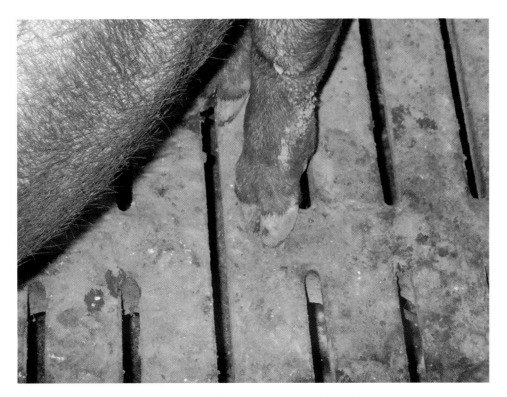

Fig. 9.10ii. Gilt with poor shoulder conformation and weak front legs.

9.10　Comments

9.10a. This type of lameness in young gilts indicates the occurrence of increased numbers of pigs with poor conformation of the legs and spine. It is a common problem in modern breeding herds that are expanding quickly and are looking to retain all their high performance hybrid pigs for more farrowings. These pigs with poor conformation that are retained for growth and fertility may have a much higher tendency to have feet and joint problems and to become lame during pregnancy or lactation. The selection of young breeding females is an important process on a breeding farm and requires the farmer to have appropriate experience and an eye for body conformation.

9.10b. These lameness and conformation problems will become more common if pigs are only selected for other factors such as high growth rates, feed conversion or for their fertility features (e.g. numbers of piglets born alive). Breeding programmes in pigs are somewhat slow processes, with the offspring of any particular mating only reaching their own entry to the breeding herd around 9 months after the mating. So it is vital that breeding farms attempt to collect as much information as possible during the mating and selection processes. This is needed to make balanced decisions on each young breeding female as to whether she should enter the breeding herd or be culled. Training materials exist on the Internet with many comparative pictures, videos and comments on the optimum body conformation for pigs.

9.11 Case Study

The farmer operated an established finisher and fattening unit, with one large older-style building, which had many smaller pens. The farmer generally went around to local markets and pig dealers in his truck to buy some pigs for the farm. These incoming pigs were generally around 25–30 kg bodyweight. These pigs were then placed into some empty pens and fed and raised until they were 120–140 kg bodyweight, for sale to local markets. Over a period of some weeks, the farmer noticed that some of the growing pigs in a few pens had a lower feed intake and were slightly lame. These pigs were lying down most of the time (Fig. 9.11i). Close inspection of the feet of these pigs indicated that they had a few small ulcers and vesicles on the sides of their feet, just above the hoof, and sometimes in between the claws (Fig. 9.11ii). These lesions were more clearly visible when the feet were washed. There did not appear to be any obvious vesicles on the face. The feet lesions seemed older in some pigs and some pigs seemed to have foot lesions that had healed.

Key Features

- Continuous flow of pigs on a smaller farm.
- Mild lameness in some growing pigs.
- Some ulcers and vesicles at the side of feet.

9.11a. What could this problem be?
9.11b. What control measures may assist the herd?

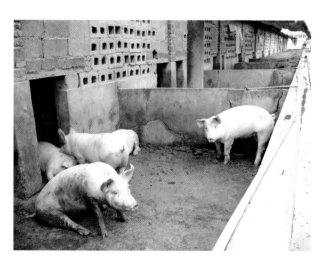

Fig. 9.11i. Groups of normal and lame pigs in older buildings.

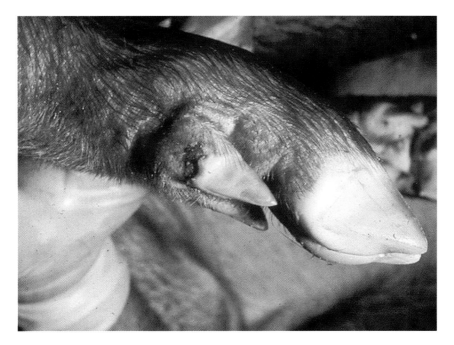

Fig. 9.11ii. Small ulcers and vesicles at the side of the foot.

9:11 Comments

9.11a. This history and the clinical signs are suggestive of the current form of swine vesicular disease (SVD) arriving on to a pig farm site. At the time of writing, this disease has been confined to southern Italy, in this mild form, for some 20 years. However, the recent experience of ASF breaking out from a small and dormant role in the global pig industry, to become a major threat to the stability of global pig farming, means that attention must be given to regional diseases, such as SVD. Because of the potential for spread of this disease and its importance in international trade, it is important to get full information in all situations that may resemble this case study. In particular, the possibility that the similar but more serious FMD may be involved must be investigated. So questions would include:

1. What recent farmed animal movements on or off the farm have occurred?
2. Are other pigs on the farm affected?
3. Do any neighbouring farms have similar problems, which may include goats, cattle or sheep?

9.11b. SVD in its current form is very mild and much less contagious than FMD. On affected farms and on dealer premises and markets, it has been difficult to eradicate because the virus is so tough and persistent. Any suspicion of SVD should lead to the farmer calling the government authorities, who may stop all movement of people and animals on and off the farm. Samples of vesicle fluid, other tissues and blood samples must be sent to designated laboratories in secure packaging for virus isolation and identification.

PART 10
Fertility Problems In Pigs

10.1 Case Study

The farmer operated a group of modern breeding farms, with a separate boar stud and artificial insemination programme. The breeder farms were in isolated areas with excellent biosecurity. Gilts were moved from one facility to another at various times for the breeding programmes. On one facility, the new gilt pigs were housed in large groups in open pens, which made handling the pigs for vaccinations and other procedures difficult. One of these groups of developing gilts was transported to another breeding farm, where they were vaccinated and mated, all within the first 2 weeks of arrival. The gestations proceeded normally, with conception rates and farrowing rates within target levels. The farmer noticed increasing numbers of litters, with normal numbers of piglets born, but with a high number of weak and stillborn (newborn piglets born dead) (Fig. 10.1i). Close inspection of the litters indicated that many of the dead piglets had been born in a mummified state (i.e. small, with dark brown, dry skin and bones) (Fig. 10.1ii). This problem eventually affected about 30% of the litters from this group of gilts. The gilts that produced these mummified litters appeared normal. The boar semen used for these gilts produced normal piglet litters in other farms.

Key Features

- Modern breeding farm with less than optimal vaccination programme.
- Numerous mummified fetuses in litters.

10.1a. What is this problem?
10.1b. What control measures may assist the herd?

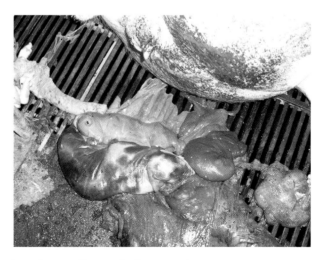

Fig. 10.1i. Abortion of mummified and stillborn piglets.

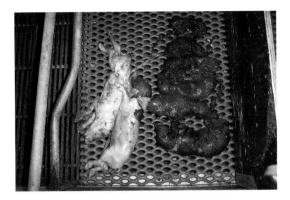

Fig. 10.1ii. Litter with many mummified piglets.

10.1 Comments

10.1a. The 'normal' sporadic and unexplained abortion rate across all pregnant pigs is approximately 1–2% of pigs that are mated and achieve a pregnancy. Therefore the finding of up to 30% of pigs with mummies, stillborns and weak piglets in this case is suggestive of an infectious agent attacking the fetuses. The routes of infection of pig fetuses by abortogenic agents such as viruses and bacteria are usually via the bloodstream following an initial infection.

The identification of numerous litters with mummified dead piglets is suspicious of porcine parvovirus (PPV) infection. PPV is a ubiquitous and persistent organism on most pig farms, often circulating in the nursery area. Early exposure of young pigs, therefore generally leads to common antibody titres and an associated herd immunity in most herds. This immunity can occur even without the use of commercial parvovirus vaccination. However, on modern pig farms in isolated areas, with or without any boars present, then pigs may lack the natural parvovirus immunity. After weaning, pigs intended for breeding are normally held in groups in single-sex pens or enclosures. Most production gilts from commercial breed lines will attain puberty and commence oestrous between 23 and 25 weeks of age. These pigs will therefore require vaccination well before possible exposure at mating times. PPV is still a common problem seen occasionally on many farms, where the parvovirus vaccination programmes are weak or badly implemented.

10.1b. It is important that all gilts are fully protected with vaccination programmes for parvovirus and other agents. Vaccine injections do not have an immediate effect and all vaccines generally take at least 3 weeks to become active. Vaccination programmes therefore need to be given well in advance of any pig movements or matings on new breeding farm areas. When farms choose to raise large groups of older finisher pigs and gilts, then it must be recognized that these pigs can be difficult for staff to handle and it means that vaccination protocols can be difficult to apply to every pig. Gilts that will be used for breeding need to be identified so that a two-dose vaccination programme can be implemented. The doses should be given 3–5 weeks apart and the second dose should be given 2 weeks before breeding.

Gilts do **NOT** have much innate immunity to breeding area infections and need plenty of preparation, good quality vaccination protocols and plenty of time for the acquired immunity to be properly established.

10.2   Case Study

The farmer operated an established breeder farm, with various older buildings. The farrowing rates and numbers born alive were at the target levels. The farmer used a complete vaccination programme for the breeding pigs. Gilts and sows were housed in small gestation and farrowing pens, with poorly drained solid-concrete floors. The farm only had a few casual staff and the floors had become damp and dirty with urine and faeces in many areas (Fig. 10.2i). In some pens, the farmer had placed wooden shavings for the pigs to lie on. The staff occasionally provided manual assistance to the sows at farrowing times. The farmer noticed that some of the sows just after farrowing were dull, depressed and reluctant to rise or suckle. These sows did not appear to be eating much. The piglets in the litters from these sows were all squealing and looking for milk. These piglets also had some diarrhoea. Close inspection of these sows showed that they had a very hot and swollen udder. The udder was firm and hard all over, not just around one teat. The udder was hot to touch, reddened and very painful, with the sow reacting instantly to the touch (Fig. 10.2ii). The sows tended to lie more on their belly, to protect the teats from the piglets. Occasionally, it was possible to express milk material from the teats, but this was a watery, clotted, grey–yellow–bloody discoloured fluid.

Key Features

- Dirty sow areas with solid floors.
- Depressed sow with no milk and piglets all hungry.
- Hot and swollen udder.

10.2a. What is this problem?
10.2b. What control measures may assist this herd?

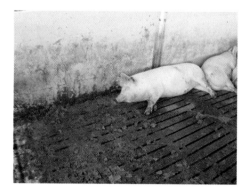

Fig. 10.2i. Sows in dirty gestation and farrowing pen areas.

10.2 Comments

10.2a. This is mastitis or inflammation of the udder. It is usually caused when bacteria from the environment enter the teat opening and ascend their way deeper into the udder and form an active infection. The specific bacteria involved can be a range of coliforms, such as *Escherichia coli* or *Klebsiella* spp., which occur commonly in pig faeces and the environment. Therefore the disease is more likely when gestation and lactation pens are not properly cleaned and when warm, moist conditions allow the bacteria

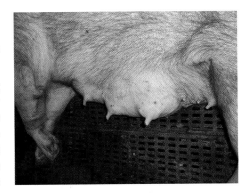

Fig. 10.2ii. A painful and swollen udder.

to accumulate. This form of overall mastitis can be compared to a more localized inflammation in a single gland, which may be due to a localized teat lesion. These localized hard lumps are often noted in one of the rear glands. It is also important to check that the condition is a full udder inflammation and not the lack of milk, known as agalactia, which is a different problem.

Functioning mammary glands of sows are vital for piglet survival and growth. The sow normally has one or two thoracic glands, four pairs of abdominal glands and one pair of inguinal glands. The front glands generally are larger and produce much more milk than the rear ones. Unlike in dogs and humans, there is no transfer of any protective materials through the placental membranes in foetal pigs. The piglet is therefore born 'naked' and requires an immediate intake of these protective materials, such as cells and antibodies, contained in the first milk of the sow, or colostrum. The colostrum should be yellow, sticky and creamy and produced for the first few days of lactation.

10.2b. The affected sow may be treated with injections and intra-mammary antibiotics and anti-inflammatory products, which will reduce both the pain and the inflammation. However, the situation is often a difficult one if the sow has a diseased udder and cannot provide milk for the current litter. The piglets therefore will need to be fostered by a healthy sow and closely observed to make sure they are receiving milk. In addition the piglets will do better if they receive treatment for diarrhoea and are kept warm and clean. The diseased sow may die even with treatment and is usually culled.

The main objective to prevent mastitis is to provide a clean and hygienic place for the sow to produce milk. The farrowing pens should be clean and disinfected and given plenty of time to dry fully, prior to entry of the sow. It is best to avoid the use of beddings such as wood shavings around the farrowing period, as these can carry many environmental bacteria. There is some debate on the value of thoroughly washing and cleaning the sows and their udders themselves prior to entry to the farrowing areas. Many farms perform this job, but it probably has the most beneficial effect if the pre-farrow sows are allowed to dry completely before they enter the hygienic farrowing areas. Keeping these pre-farrowed sows in well-cleaned crates to maintain the level of hygiene is very important.

10.3   Case Study

The farmer operated a large breeding farm and had been busy expanding the gilt herd and introducing new modern lines of breeding pigs. There was a mixture of new and old lines of gilts and sows. The farmer had a successful mating programme and groups of gilts mated with excellent boars with normal farrowing rates. The successful breeding programme also led to an increasing number of piglets born alive in each litter. These piglets were born into clean and modern farrowing areas. The farmer had been focused on the breeding programme and had not changed any of the various diets given to the different stages of these breeding pigs. The farmer noticed that around the time of farrowing and lactation, the udders on some gilts had become small and inactive (Fig. 10.3i), so that the newly born piglets had difficulty finding any colostrum or milk. Close inspection showed that the udder of these gilts was small, firm and inactive, with very little or no milk production. The udder was very firm at the place where the udder attached to the abdomen. The udder was not particularly painful. In some affected gilts, there was fluid build-up noticeable at the rear of the udder and between the back legs. These affected gilts generally appeared to be of a smaller overall size and were thin and listless. This udder problem seemed to occur at different times, either soon after birth or at around 1 week after birth. In the gilts that were affected soon after birth, there were a large number of piglets in the litter. In the gilts affected 1 week after birth, there were only a few piglets in the litter (Fig. 10.3ii).

Key Features

- Gestation and lactation diets are variable.
- Udder tissue is poorly developed.

10.3a. What is this problem?
10.3b. What control measures may assist the herd?

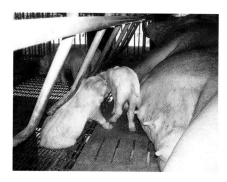

Fig. 10.3i. Thin gilt with small udder and many piglets.

10.3 Comments

10.3a. This is agalactia or lack of milk production. It is seen primarily in gilts and is often recognized in the period immediately leading up to and immediately following farrowing. The main reason for a failure of udder tissue to develop is inadequate nutrition during the period of udder development and lactation. This may occur due to errors in feed rations and lactation diets with a limited or insufficient protein: energy ratio, in the large modern breeds of pigs. This will be more prominent in gilts or small sows that deliver a large litter. If the feed mill produces low-density forms of diets, the gilts may have extreme difficulty in consuming sufficient feed to provide for both their own maintenance growth and for the milk for their litter. These pigs will begin to use their own body fat to make up any deficiency, so will appear thin and fail to produce milk. Poor appetite and poor milk production in breeder pigs is a major global problem in pig farming.

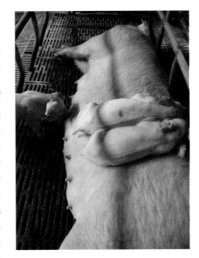

Fig. 10.3ii. Gilt with small udder and few piglets.

A related problem is where milk is produced initially, but where agalactia develops a week or so after farrowing. The litter of piglets will start well but will taper off without milk. This can again occur due to poor nutrition of the gilt. It can also occur if the litter is small – the main stimulus for continued milk production is the removal of milk by the suckling piglets. Therefore, if there is no litter or there are only a few weak piglets, then there will be insufficient stimulus to produce milk and agalactia will result. This type of agalactia will occur if there are few piglets in a litter, which may be due to diseases or other losses among the piglets.

10.3b. The affected sows and gilts are often culled (after weaning), because it can be very difficult to get them back to a fully fattened nutritional status, with full milk production. The poor appetite of gilts is a major problem in modern pig farming, so various steps are suggested to encourage breeder pigs to eat sufficient feed around the farrowing period. Various designs of feeder equipment may encourage gilts and sows to be active and eat more. Some designs allow the sows to feed throughout the day or at least two to three times per day. It is vital that sows have plenty of fresh drinking water throughout the lactation period. Flavoured feeds may be considered to improve palatability, or feed may be provided in a more concentrated and wet-mash format. This need for specialized feeding phases needs to be discussed clearly between farmers and their feed mills. Feed-mill operators will generally aim for producing only a small number of high-volume diets, which may not be suitable for all farmers.

Gilts housed in groups need to be checked to ensure that all pigs are receiving adequate feed intakes. The use of electronic sow feeding (ESF) systems may assist this type of feeding programme.

10.4 Case Study

The farmer operated a system of breeder pig farms, with on-site boars, within an agricultural area that also had numerous rice plantations (Fig. 10.4i). These rice-growing areas had numerous waterbirds and mosquito populations, and these insects seemed most active at twilight during the late spring and early summer months. The farmer had recently been expanding the breeding herd, with introductions and breeding of many new female pigs into the herd. The vaccination programme was not fully active for the expanding breeding herd. In the middle and end of the summer period, the farmer noticed that the abortion rate among the pregnant female pigs rose from a normal rate of 2% up to 20%. Close inspection indicated that this was due to an increased number of late-term abortions and stillbirths (Fig. 10.4ii), with a few mummified fetuses. The newborn piglets that were born alive in some litters seemed weak and inactive. Some of these newborn piglets also had convulsions and tremors, with many piglet deaths in the first week of their life. All of the affected sows and the other female pigs in the breeding herd appeared normal and ate normally.

Key Features

- Farms located in rice-growing areas.
- Numerous litters with late-term abortions and stillbirths in the summer.

10.4a. What is this problem?
10.4b. What control measures may assist the herd?

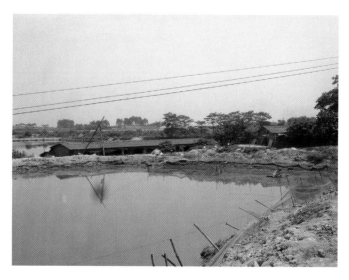

Fig. 10.4i. Pig farms in a rice-growing area.

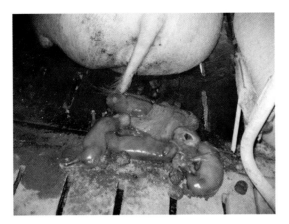

Fig. 10.4ii. Stillborn piglets in late-term abortions.

10.4   Comments

10.4a. The identification of numerous litters with dead piglets is suspicious of Japanese encephalitis (JE) virus infection. When a female pig is exposed to JE during gestation, then the litter will be affected. The diagnosis should be supported by tests for the virus on blood and serum samples from the pigs. A high titre for JE virus should be present to confirm the case. However, in many areas, this diagnosis is complicated by antibodies from vaccination or previous exposure. Testing the piglets is not usually helpful, because the sow has usually cleared the virus by the time an affected litter is born.

This disease currently occurs throughout the temperate and tropical regions of East Asia. It is an insect-borne virus, transmitted to animals when they are bitten by the carrier insect. For JE, the main insect involved is the mosquito, *Culex tritaeniorhynchus*, which breeds in rice paddies and connecting canals, and is active at twilight. The virus circulates in these insects and also in wading waterbirds that are common in rice fields. In the more temperate regions of East Asia, the JE season usually begins in May and ends in October. Waterfowl are infected when mosquitoes appear in late spring, then pigs are infected later. In tropical regions of East Asia, the JE virus circulates all year in mosquitoes, birds and pigs. However, peaks of JE disease may occur following the rainy season or irrigation periods that enhance local mosquitoes. When boars are bitten and infected by an infected mosquito, the virus may then appear in the semen, and so further transmission can occur to the inseminated female pigs.

10.4b. Prevention measures that pig farmers can apply include measures to eliminate potential mosquito breeding areas, such as standing pools of water around pig sheds. The control of JE requires the use of protective vaccines for pigs and humans. Housing the pigs in sheds with insect screens can be partially protective, particularly during outbreaks. Peak mosquito-biting activity is usually from dusk to dawn. The use of fans inside buildings is helpful, as mosquitoes do not fly well in strong winds. The walls may also be sprayed with insecticides. Insect repellents can help protect individual animals. The presence of modern pig farming in an agricultural area therefore does not necessarily increase the general risk of infection.

10.5   Case Study

The farmer operated an older-style breeder pig farm located in a cold and hilly region (Fig. 10.5i). There were various old sheds for housing pigs and several open pens used for outdoor farm areas. The farmer used these open outdoor areas for raising groups of active boars and various other female pig breeding groups. The region had various populations of wild and feral pigs in nearby woods. The health of the farm pigs was generally good, with an excellent vaccination programme. The female pigs appeared to come into heat normally, and matings proceeded normally, using the outdoor farm boars. However, over a period of months, the farmer noticed that the farrowing rate and the conception rate were decreasing. Many female pigs returned to heat 30–45 days after each breeding date. Some other mated pigs were apparently pregnant when tested at 30 days after mating, but then failed to farrow (Fig. 10.5ii). Only a few aborted piglet materials were found and many females failed to deliver any form of litter. Close inspection confirmed these records and noted the lack of late-term abortions. It was also noted that several of the sows, which had failed to farrow, showed excess discharges of mucus and bloody materials from their vulva. Some of these sows appeared slightly dull and were eating slowly. One or two of the boars on the farm appeared to have lumps at the top of their testicles.

Key Features

- Older-style farm with outdoor access.
- Reproductive problems in early pregnancy.

10.5a. What is this problem?
10.5b. What control measures may assist the herd?

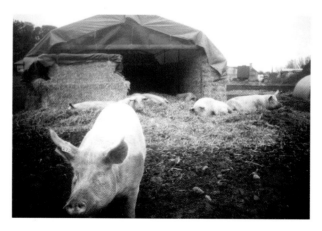

Fig. 10.5i. Older-style breeder farm with open areas in a colder region.

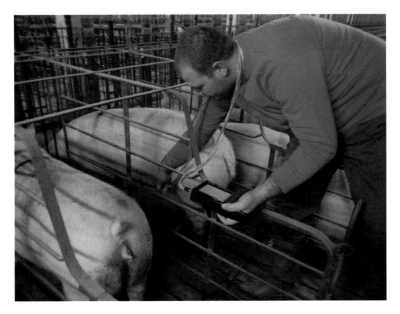

Fig. 10.5ii. Pregnancy testing for return to heat and failure to farrow.

10.5 Comments

10.5a. The key features in this case are suspicious of porcine brucellosis, caused by the bacterium *Brucella suis*. This disease is not common in modern pig farms and is now mainly seen in remote outdoor farms in colder climates. Female pigs infected with brucellosis will show various forms of infertility, with returns to oestrous and abortions in the early or middle parts of pregnancy. The infection occurs more commonly in wild and feral pigs. In some cases, the actual interaction of wild and domestic pigs and disease transmission can be direct, including the possibility that pigs may mate with or even consume abortion materials from local wild or feral pigs.

Brucellosis is a form of venereal disease, that is the boars are infected and their semen is positive, so they will infect the female pigs at the time of mating, causing the reproductive problems in early pregnancy. Only occasional pigs will show further signs, such as the vulva discharge, or inflammation of the testicles or sperm cord and epididymis. The diagnosis can be confirmed by special blood tests for *Brucella*, such as the Rose Bengal test and the bacteria may be cultured from any aborted piglets that are found in an outbreak.

10.5b. There are no vaccines for porcine brucellosis and in many situations the infected herd should be slaughtered with appropriate compensation. *B. suis* is considered a zoonosis (a disease that can be transmitted from animals to people) so protective gloves should be worn when coming into contact with blood, disposing of placental tissue and dead pigs.

10.6   Case Study

The farmer operated a large, established breeder and production farm system, with various farm sites. The farm was located in a temperate climate area with hot summers (Fig. 10.6i) and cold winters. The farmer had a well-run boar stud, which used good artificial insemination techniques throughout the year. The farm had contracts with local processors to supply them with finisher pigs in certain numbers each month. Over some years, the farmer noticed that he always had problems providing enough pigs for these contracts in the months of March through to June. This failure of pig supply was traced back to a lack of piglets being born in the months of October through to January. The records of the breeder farms were examined. Across all of the breeder farms, a mixture of reproductive problems was contributing to this lack of piglets in these winter months. The problems therefore related to attempts at breeding female pigs in the summer and autumn months of July through to October. The number of gilts and young sows that were noted to be in oestrous and mated in the autumn months was low. The breeding pigs were often kept indoors in poorly lit rooms in this period (Fig. 10.6ii). It was suggested that many of these pigs had failed to cycle in these summer and autumn months. Many other pigs were mated but returned to oestrous later. Many pigs that did become pregnant at this time had abortions in later pregnancy. The overall result was that the farrowing rates of the herds were therefore 10–20% lower than expected, during the months of October through to January.

Key Features

- Reduced farrowing rate in autumn and early winter months.
- Numerous reproductive problems in late summer contributing to the overall problem.

10.6a. What is this problem?
10.6b. What control measures may assist the herd?

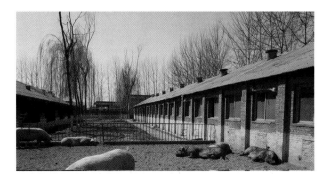

Fig. 10.6i. Inactive breeding pigs in hot weather.

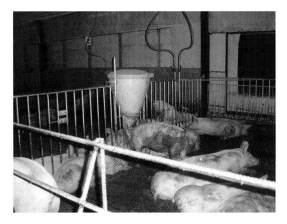

Fig. 10.6ii. Inactive breeding pigs in dark rooms in autumn.

10.6 Comments

10.6a. The identification of seasonal drops in farrowing rate is suspicious of seasonal infertility. There are generally two main components to seasonal infertility – summer infertility and autumn infertility – with slightly different causes. However, these two problems can run continually on the same farm.

Summer infertility is due to various factors associated with hot temperatures inside sheds or outdoors. The effects of hot weather on breeder female pigs include a reduced appetite among the gilts and sows, which will negatively impact on the onset of the subsequent oestrous, ovulation rates and conception. Hot temperatures will also reduce boar and sow mating activity. Hot temperatures can also lead to loss of a pregnancy, due to heat stress and the need for maintenance of suitable core body temperatures.

Autumn infertility is due to the many hormonal changes in the pig experiencing a rapid decrease in day length at this time. Any sow house exposed to natural lighting can be vulnerable to this rapid decrease in day length. These associated hormonal changes seem to reduce overall reproductive system activity in females.

10.6b. Many pig farms develop procedures to cool their pigs in summer. Sheds should have adequate insulation and ventilation systems. Water sprays can be applied to the pigs, the floors or the outside roof, for evaporative cooling effects. Female pigs should always be given free access to cold drinking water.

Regarding autumn infertility, for the breeder herd kept indoors, lighting levels can be controlled. A day length of 14–16 h of lighting can be provided from mid- to late summer for the breeding pigs and may offset the reduction in natural light patterns. The judgement of sufficient extra light for the pigs is considered to be at the level required to read a newspaper in the sheds. It is also considered useful to increase the contact of female pigs with boars, to stimulate further cycle activity in the autumn.

Seasonal infertility is a common and serious problem, with no simple solutions to the reduced farrowing rates. The management response in many farms is often to basically just increase the total number of pigs mated through the summer and autumn, leading to the target number of farrowings and production pigs. So the farm may reduce the culling of older sows and increase the number of gilts and their matings through this summer and autumn period.

10.7 Case Study

The farmer operated an established breeder farm, with some older buildings, housing different groups of females and boars. The farmer kept good records of the female pigs and the breeding programmes. The farmer was expanding the breeder herd and had placed various large groups of gilts and sows in some open and overcrowded pens in the older buildings (Fig. 10.7i). Many new gilts in these groups were being selected for the breeding herd and initial matings. The farm staff then performed a combination of artificial insemination (AI) and natural mating techniques. The AI semen came from a distant boar stud and the semen deliveries for the farm arrived in old trucks. The natural matings occurred in busy mating pens in one of the older buildings. The boars used for these natural matings were housed in older-building areas (Fig. 10.7ii). Over the summer months, the farm pregnancy testing indicated that the conception rate was low, at only 80%, with the resulting farrowing rate also low, at 75%. Close inspection of the breeding records indicated that many of the non-pregnant gilts and sows were not 'holding' their matings, with these gilts and sows showing a normal oestrous 21 days after the previous oestrous and mating. These were classified as regular returns to service and not pregnant. The problem was considered to be worse in the gilts.

Key Features

- Busy breeder farm.
- High rate of return to service.

10.7a. What is this problem?
10.7b. What control measures may assist the herd?

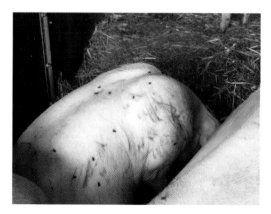

Fig. 10.7i. Gilts with fighting wounds in overcrowded pens.

10.7 Comments

10.7a. The identification of drops in conception rate is suspicious of poor breeding farm techniques. This farm problem may be due to various interacting issues.

After weaning, pigs are normally held in groups in single-sex pens or enclosures. Most production gilts from commercial breed lines will attain puberty and commence oestrous between 23 and 25 weeks of age. The production and activity of ovarian follicles will be reduced where gilts and sows are kept in over-crowded groups of thin, busy fighting sows and mating pens. One important result of keeping gilts and sows in large groups in open pens is that many can become thin and stressed, with traumatic injuries and reduced access to feeders, due to 'aggressor' females. These aggressor pigs will commence and deter-minedly continue strong fighting using their tusks to slash at flanks of other pigs in the group. The bullying

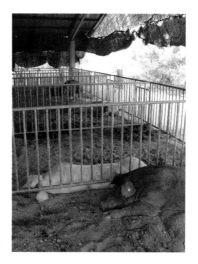

Fig. 10.7ii. Inactive breeding boar pigs in hot weather.

aggressor will also lead to the other pigs losing full access to feeders and waterers, which can lead to gilts with poor body condition and becoming dehydrated. These thin gilts may have noticeable flank wounds, with wounds at other locations such as the vulva or ear, and tail biting may also be evident. The main result in the breeder herd will be a reduction in the conception rate, particularly in the gilts.

A further issue in low conception rate and poor breeding farm techniques is related to the housing of boars and sows in the summer months. Natural mating with boars is less active in the hot summer months, with less effective mating, particularly if the mating pens are overcrowded. Any time the temperature is over 27°C and humidity higher than 50%, the volume and quality of semen will be affected. Boars must be housed in a way to keep them as cool as possible. The effect of heat on boar semen quality can last 6–7 weeks until it recovers. There may also be a deterioration of boar semen in transit in hot weather, from a stud to a breeder farm.

10.7b. The breeder farm must look to improve the condition and stress levels of the gilts up to mating. The management of pens and mating protocols must enable the pigs to feel comfortable. The use of stalls to house gilts can improve their conception rates. Gilts themselves are growing animals and not having ready access to feed and water will impact their future productivity in the herd.

The AI service must be checked to make sure that semen quality is maintained with active sperm from the stud to the farm. Boar semen must be carefully transported in appro-priate maintenance fluid (extension fluids) at the appropriate temperature. Semen used for AI must be kept at 17°C during transportation and usage. Any variation in temperature up or down will affect the quality and longevity of the semen and affect conception rates.

10.8   Case Study

The farmer operated a large breeder and production farm, in a region with many other local pig farms nearby. The farmer maintained a variety of pig breeds and cross-breeding programmes. He usually purchased some new gilt replacements for these different lines of pigs, every 6 months. There was also a variety of boars on the farm, to match the different breeding programmes. Over a period of several months, the farmer noticed a marked variability and general decrease in the farrowing rate and the number of piglets born alive. The mating procedures, conception rates and early pregnancy seemed to be normal. The main cause of the low farrowing rate seemed to be an increase in the number of late-term abortions, stillborn piglets and with some of the dead piglets born in a mummified state. Close inspection of the breeding farm records over the past 2 years showed some repeating patterns evident. For periods of around 2 months, 5–20% of farrowing pigs had abortions and stillbirths, with numerous piglets born dead (Fig. 10.8i). Typically in litters born with 10–14 piglets, only one or two piglets would be born alive. After the 2 month period, the number of piglets born alive would slowly increase back to normal. The same sows that had previously had litters with numbers of piglets born alive (NBA) of one or two, then had normal litters with 10, 12 or more normal piglets at the next litter. Then 6 months after this period of normal figures, once again the abortions and stillbirths started again, for another 2 month period. These cycles of abortions were noted consistently over the past 2 years at least, leading to an average rate of only nine piglets born alive per litter over that period. The affected sows sometimes appeared lethargic and some had dull blue to purple coloration of their ears (Fig. 10.8ii). At examination of the abortions and stillborn piglets, the farmer and the veterinarian noticed that some 2 cm long haemorrhages were evident in the umbilical cords and that some piglets had an increase in fluid in their chest cavity.

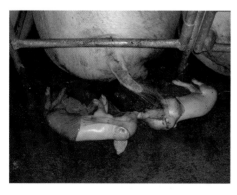

Fig. 10.8i. Many stillborn and dead piglets in litters.

Key Features

- Active breeder farm in pig-dense area.
- Recurring periods of reproductive problems.
- Numerous abortions and stillborn fetuses in litters.

10.8a. What is this problem?
10.8b. What control measures may assist this herd?

10.8 Comments

10.8a. The identification of recurring patterns of late-term abortions and stillbirths with numerous litters with dead piglets is suspicious of PRRS virus. This is the most common and important infection in pigs across the world of pig farming. There are two main strains of PRRS, the European strain and the American strain; the latter one tends to have a much bigger impact on pig farms. Many farms in Asia are infected with both strains. The PRRS virus has a number of special qualities that have made it the major virus affecting pigs. It consists of a single strand of nucleic acid, which

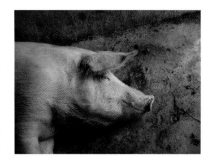

Fig. 10.8ii. Lethargic sow with dull-blue-to-purple-coloured ears.

can change easily and make new strains. These new PRRS strains can appear on a single farm, or they can arrive on the wind or when new pigs are introduced. It is a very common infection so introduction of new weaners, gilts and boars from other farms is a high risk for bringing in new strains. The semen of boars can remain positive for PRRS for 3 months and spread the infection further among the sows. There is often cross-transmission of PRRS between age groups. In farms where weaner pigs are located near the breeder pigs, then the weaners can continually send new infections to the breeding herd. PRRS virus has proved difficult to control, particularly in areas where there are many pig farms in nearby areas. Because there are many strains, and new strains are continually evolving, then having a recent outbreak of PRRS does not provide any immunity to the next PRRS virus entry and disease outbreak. It is therefore a common and ongoing problem.

10.8b. It has proved possible to eradicate PRRS infections from breeding farms, by operating a closed herd and waiting for immunity to develop in the sows. If the breeding herd is kept completely closed (i.e. isolated and no introductions occur) then the infected sows will eventually become immune and stop shedding the virus. This clearance process takes about 2 months. After some months, these immune sows can then be inseminated with PRRS-negative semen and produce PRRS-negative litters of piglets. These piglets may be raised to become PRRS-negative nursery and grower pigs, if they are also kept fully isolated from other pigs. This technique of control of PRRS infections is reasonably well understood, but the main problem is prevention of new infections. For a farm system to use this process, requires good isolation of the farms and prevention of new infections in the future from the outside as well as preventing the circulation of viruses within the herd. It is therefore difficult to follow this programme in an area with many other pig farms nearby.

The control of PRRS therefore often relies on vaccines. Various PRRS vaccines are available. The modified live PRRS vaccines have been useful at providing some protection to pigs, which may be exposed to PRRS virus strains similar to the ones present in the vaccine. It is often important to establish what strain of PRRS virus is on the pig farm. This usually requires the use of PCR tests. The vaccine should be applied to non-pregnant gilts or sows at the time of mating.

10.9   Case Study

The farmer operated a large modern breeder farm and some other business enterprises. The farmer had recently employed an inexperienced breeder farm manager and many of the farm staff were casual labour. The oestrous detection and mating procedures were generally well conducted and the boar semen was good quality. The number of piglets in each litter born seemed normal and only 1% or 2% of sows were noted with late-term abortions. The farm records were not complete, but the farmer had noticed that the number of litters born and the farrowing rate had dropped to 75–80% of matings, rather than the target level of 90% (Fig. 10.9i). The farrowing rate among the sows and gilts had stayed at this level of 75–80% over the past months. The records also indicated that the conception rate, that is the number of pigs reported to be pregnant, when checked by ultrasound image technique at 30 days of pregnancy (Fig. 10.9ii), was at an acceptable level of 90%. The problem was therefore considered to be a low farrowing rate, in the presence of normal conception. Some of the more experienced farm staff suggested that many of the sows had appeared to be slightly dull and ill over the past months.

Key Features

- Normal conception rate apparent.
- Low farrowing rate without an abortion problem.

10.9a. What are the likely problems and how can they be confirmed?

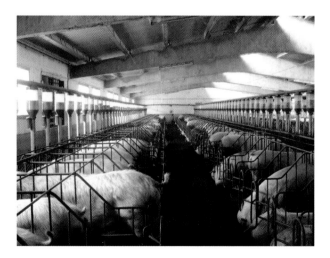

Fig. 10.9i. Large modern breeder with low farrowing rates.

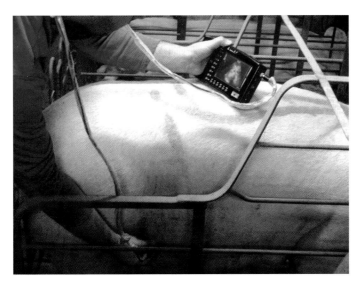

Fig. 10.9ii. Farm worker checking pregnancy diagnosis.

10.9 Comments

10.9a. The likely problems here involve a reduced farrowing rate due to poor management of the breeding herd. This may involve the areas of sow retention and replacements, health checks and pregnancy diagnosis.

First, the records of the farm may show that the matings and pregnancy levels among the sows are actually normal, but that the inexperienced manager and his team are culling and removing too many sows while they are pregnant and in the gestation area. Farm management must choose the priority for culling sows and the best times to cull sows. Sows may be culled for various reasons such as: (i) lameness; (ii) poor conformation; (iii) poor appetite; (iv) aggression behaviours; and (v) tail-biting lesions. If many of these animals are culled during pregnancy, then the farrowing rate will appear to be reduced. The diagnosis of this kind of management issue requires careful inspection of sow numbers and reasons and dates of culling.

A second reason for a reduced farrowing rate is when a low to medium health problem occurs among the sows in gestation. In modern pig farms, this type of health problem may be swine influenza or other moderate and common virus infection. The sows may show only a few signs of coughing and only appear lethargic with a low appetite. These infections may be diagnosed by testing the blood of the sows.

The third reason for an apparent reduction in farrowing rate occurs when the staff who perform the pregnancy diagnosis are not trained and do not use appropriate equipment. In this situation, the pregnancy diagnosis staff may be reporting a normal conception rate. But this is false information and many of the pigs are in fact not pregnant, due to poor mating practices. For example, the oestrous detection and checking is not performed properly, perhaps only once per day. This can lead to mating and inseminations occurring at an inappropriate stage in the oestrous cycle of the sow. There may be many occasions when the mating and semen and other factors required to start a pregnancy are not optimal. The diagnosis of this kind of management issue requires farm managers to be skilled at detecting staff failures.

10.10   Case Study

The farmer operated a breeder farm system with some cross-breed hybrid lines in multiplier and production herds and a few different pure-breed grandparent lines in nucleus herds. The breeder farm system consisted of several farm sites, some with older-style sheds and some with new modern purpose-built breeder pig facilities. The cross-breed hybrid pig lines were generally housed on the sites with older-style sheds, whereas the valuable grandparent lines were housed on the sites with modern sheds. The older-style farrowing sheds tended to have only a few casual labour staff with an older manager (Fig. 10.10i). For the management of pure-breed lines in the nucleus herds, the farmer was self-taught in pig breeding and had retained many of these old pure-breed pigs for several years. He had devised a closed-herd system and used various mating formula among these nucleus sows and boars. Across the farm system, the conception rate was considered acceptable at over 90%. The farrowing rate was also acceptable at over 85%, with few abortions. However, across the farm system, the numbers of pigs born alive in each litter was considered very low, with records indicating only eight or nine normal piglets born alive on both the older-style and the modern farm sites. The problem therefore appeared to be small litter sizes of viable pigs (Fig. 10.10ii).

Key Features

- Normal conception and farrowing rates.
- Numbers of piglets born alive are low with small litters of viable pigs.

10.10a. What is this problem?
10.10b. What control measures may assist the herd?

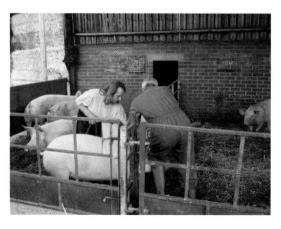

Fig. 10.10i. Older-style breeding units.

10.10 Comments

10.10a. The occurrence of small litter sizes is usually due to management problems in the breeder farm system. The neonatal litter is often the focus of interest in normal farrowings. The first problem on the older-style farrowing areas with hybrid sows is likely to be a failure to properly record the status of piglets at birth. Most sows give birth at night and if staff activity is low, then many litters may only be examined several hours after birth has finished. It is possible that many young piglets that were born alive and healthy may be crushed by the sow, and so are overlay cases. The staff failure can therefore be to misclassify these dead piglet cases as being stillborn cases, making the number of viable piglets per litter (NBA) look low, whereas in fact it may be near normal.

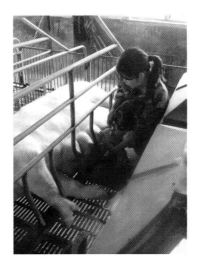

Fig. 10.10ii. Small litter size of viable piglets of pure-breed pigs.

The low litter size problem in the various lines of pure-breed pigs is likely to be an excess of older sows that are mated in a haphazard way, without a proper genetics programme involving scientific checking of hybrid lines, with matings of non-relatives. If pure-breed pig matings are performed in this non-scientific genetics programme, then small litter size is often a noticeable outcome.

10.10b. The experience of most pig farms is that staff in the farrowing areas must have good attention to detail and a proper maternal instinct to looking after the newborn piglets. One of the most useful interventions a pig breeder farm can make is to establish good staff in the farrowing houses at night-times when most litters are born. Farms should routinely collect accurate data on the numbers of piglets born alive and dead, as this will have a major impact on farm profitability and breeding programmes. Most piglets that are born dead (i.e. a pre-parturition death) are known as stillborn and are recognized by the presence of dried mucus over the body and soft unworn hooves. On dissection, these piglets will have un-inflated lungs, an empty stomach and meconium in the upper respiratory tract. Mummies are included as a separate category within the overall category of piglets born dead. The largest category of neonatal piglet deaths in normal farm situations is often that of a piglet in good body condition that is found dead in the first few days of its life. The death of these piglets is usually due to suffocation from being overlain and crushed by the mothering sow.

The proper development of the genetics of a breeding programme is a scientific exercise and the farmer should take appropriate technical advice in this area. Most pig farms would look for technical advice in the areas of health and veterinary issues, genetics, nutrition and environmental waste management. Many larger farms may employ professional staff in these areas, but smaller farms can use appropriate consultants on a regular basis.

10.11 Case Study

The farmer operated a medium-size breeder farm. The farmer liked to have a range of different lines and breeds of pigs, which he purchased from some small local breeder farms. The farmer regularly maintained various boars and grandparent female pigs from these different lines, for the mating programmes. The farm had good records and the conception rate and farrowing rates were generally in an acceptable range. The number of piglets born alive per litter was also normal. However, the mortality among piglets was higher than normal, with some litters having a few extra deaths or piglet removals before the weaning stage. Close inspection indicated that many piglets in different litters were born alive, but were born with different forms of physical defects (Fig. 10.11i). There were three main forms of physical defects in this farm. First, some male piglets appeared to only have one testicle in their scrotum, with the other testicle remaining inside the abdomen. This condition is known as a cryptorchid piglet (Fig. 10.11ii). The second form of defect was apparent in some male and female piglets, which had a blind and blocked anus, with no clear opening. This condition is known as atresia ani. Thirdly, some female piglets appeared to only have very small vulvas and few teats. At autopsy, when these female pigs were examined, their internal uterus and ovary were tiny and difficult to locate. This condition is known as intersex, or hermaphroditism.

Key Features

- Various birth defects reaching a noticeable level.

10.11a. What is this problem?
10.11b. What control measures may assist the herd?

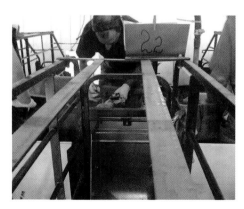

Fig. 10.11i. Examination of newborn piglets for birth defects.

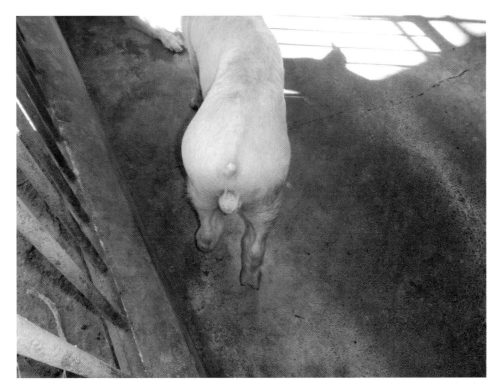

Fig. 10.11ii. Cryptorchid male piglet.

10.11 Comments

10.11a. The occurrence of birth defects suggests a mismatch among the pigs in the genetic programme causing an increase in genetic mutations in the unborn piglet and subsequent birth defects. It usually occurs when pigs that are in the same family are mated together. Matings among relatives leads to a greater likelihood of mismatched DNA in the offspring and the introduction of a slight DNA defect will lead to these piglets being born alive, but with some inherited and congenital defect.

Cryptorchid and intersex defects are reasonably common among pigs. They can be disruptive to breeding programmes if the pigs are left intact in the breeding herd. Atresia ani is quite rare but is always fatal to the piglet. A wide range of other congenital defects have been reported in piglets, such as skin defects, but these will vary in prevalence and fade away if the affected lines of pigs are side-lined.

10.11b. The control measure is simply to note and avoid the particular mating combination of these pigs, which produced these defects.

10.12 Case Study

The farmer operated a large and modern breeder farm, with numerous sows from modern commercial hybrid lines. These pigs showed excellent growth rates, lean meat percentage and feed conversion in the production phases. The breeder farm was in an isolated location with good biosecurity and low levels of health problems. The farmer was expanding the overall breeding herd by increasing the numbers of gilts for mating. These gilts were selected from within the groups of younger production female pigs and then raised to the first mating stage in separate buildings away from other pigs. After some staff changes, this job of gilt selection and maintenance was performed by a young manager (Fig. 10.12i). The semen used for the gilts was considered of good quality and fertility. Over the next few months, the farmer noticed that the conception rate in these groups of pigs was low. The problem seemed worse in the gilts, with conception rates of only 80%, compared with a target level of 95%. Close inspection indicated that the staff were well trained and capable of heat detection, but the gilts were not showing strong or clear signs of oestrous heat (Fig. 10.12ii). The low conception rate was due to low numbers of gilts that were displaying oestrous, with many attempted matings and inseminations that were not successful. Many of the gilts in the mating pens appeared to be slightly small and in thin condition.

Key Features

- Gilt pigs do not display proper oestrous and have low conception rates.

10.12a. What is this problem?
10.12b. What control measures may assist the herd?

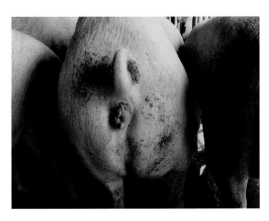

Fig. 10.12i. Gilt with properly developed vulva in oestrous, one of the clear signs of oestrous heat.

10.12 Comments

10.12a. The low conception rate is due to a failure of proper reproductive system development in gilts. After weaning, pigs are normally held in groups in single-sex pens or enclosures. Most production gilts from commercial breed lines will attain puberty and commence oestrous between 23 and 25 weeks of age. However, this onset of active puberty will be slow and delayed if the gilts are not in the best body condition. Thin and poor-growing female pigs will always show poor breeding performance. Besides the body weight of the female pig, the amount of body fat

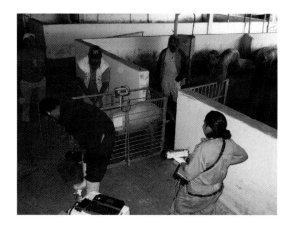

Fig. 10.12ii. Selection of gilts for proper weight and backfat.

on the female pig is also vital for proper development. Most reproductive hormones are synthesized from body fats and females with adequate or greater amounts of body fat will have better reproductive performance. The usual figures are that gilts should be at least 130 kg bodyweight at around 220 days old (31 weeks of age). They should have at least 20 mm of backfat at the P2 level. P2 is the level of the body at the head of the last rib and 6.5 cm from the midline. The selection of modern lines of pigs for a high percentage of lean meat, can have the side effect that the female pigs have insufficient back and body fat for proper reproductive performance. The other factor that is important for proper development of gilts is boar stimulation. The learned and innate oestrous behaviours needed for proper matings of gilts are enhanced if gilts are raised with periods of direct contact with male pigs. In many farms, this can be achieved by placement of vasectomized boars among the groups of gilts.

10.12b. Gilt selection is a difficult and important job and requires an experienced team looking at: (i) pig weights; (ii) pig backfat data; and (iii) other factors, such as teat numbers, vulva and leg conformation. This is in addition to gilt preparation requirements in vaccinations and proper nutrition levels.

The onset of heat in pigs can also be enhanced by judicious use of artificial hormonal preparations:

- For non-cycling gilts – Prostaglandin PG 600 is a hormone combination of PMSG (pregnant mare serum gonadotropin) and HcG (human chorionic gonadotropin) which stimulates the follicles on the ovaries to grow and produce oestrogen, which will make the gilt express oestrus (standing heat) about 4–6 days after the injection. It cannot be used in gilts that already have heat cycles.
- For gilts that have heat cycles – Active progesterone-like hormones may be given orally to synchronize the oestrous cycling of gilts. These products are fed for several consecutive days then oestrous and breeding can occur at 1 week after withdrawal of the hormone.

10.13   Case Study

The farmer operated a large breeder farm system with different and new lines of commercial breeding pigs. The gilts and sows were kept in large groups in open pens and the space was limited in some pens of the rapidly growing and vigorous gilts. Most production gilts from these commercial breed lines were coming up to the age of puberty at 23–25 weeks of age. The changes in breeding programmes in some lines of pigs led to an increase in the mixing of pigs among these groups of gilt pigs. Some pigs were placed in pens with an electronic feeding-system area (Fig. 10.13i). Many groups of these pubertal and older pigs showed hostile activity to the farm worker attendants who entered the pens. The farmer noticed an increased number of thin sows and gilts, many with noticeable wounds on their flanks (Fig. 10.13ii). Some pigs also had wounds at other body locations such as the vulva or ears. This led to some pigs with swollen bloody ears (known as aural haematoma) and in some pigs the ear tags were torn off. The main problem was agitation and wounds on the flanks of the younger gilts reaching puberty, with loss of body condition and the loss of reproductive performance.

Key Features

- Gilt pigs raised in same-sex groups in open pens.
- Some gilts show wounds on their flanks.

10.13a. What is this problem?
10.13b. What control measures may assist the herd?

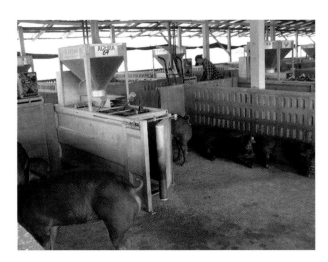

Fig. 10.13i. Gilts housed in pens with electronic feeding systems.

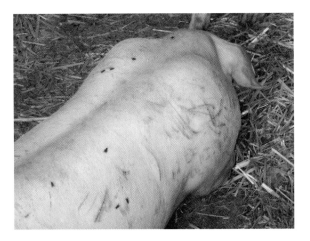

Fig. 10.13ii. Groups of gilt pigs with wounds on their flanks.

10.13 Comments

10.13a. This problem is the visible results of gilts and sows fighting, when raised in groups. Traumatic injuries among these groups of pubertal gilts (or boars) will include aggressive slashes and bites to areas of pen-mates such as the flanks, vulva and tails, particularly using their canine teeth or tusks. These aggressor pigs will commence and determinedly continue strong fighting using their tusks to slash at flanks of other pigs in the group. Skin abrasions along the flanks will quickly become evident and may become numerous, deep and severe. The bullying aggressor will also lead to other pigs losing full access to feeders and waterers, which can lead to pubertal pigs noted with poor body condition and being dehydrated.

It is strongly urged for all farm workers who must perform pen entry in these situations, to have a companion standing outside, who can assist if necessary. Also, each pen, walkway or enclosure should be entered with an escape route available if required, particularly for entry into pens or structures containing these pubertal and mature boars or sows. The wall of the pen, or the fence of any outdoor enclosure, should be low enough to leap over, perhaps in a Superman-style take-off movement.

10.13b. Many pig farm systems use a variety of methods to reduce the impact of this gilt aggression problem. Pigs reaching puberty may be housed in single animal stalls, which will obviously limit any pig-to-pig aggression. However, stalls are expensive to construct and greatly limit the pig's room for movement, with the consequent development of boredom, shoulder sores and leg weakness.

Pigs raised in groups in pens may be placed into large pens that have been designed with a row of open-access stalls allowing any pig or human under attack to retreat. Pigs raised in groups in pens may also be placed into pens with partially protected areas, such as pens that contain vertical rubber mats, which act to separate and protect pigs within groups. The use of electronic sow feeder systems theoretically allows all pigs in a group to obtain full access to feed and water. However, these systems are also expensive to construct and can lead to loss of access to feed, if any fault occurs, such as an electrical fault or loss of a radio ear tag.

PART 11
Skin and Muscle Problems in Pigs

11.1   Case Study

The farmer operated an older breeder, nursery and finisher pig farm system that had been established for many years. The farmer occasionally purchased new replacement breeder stock from nearby farms. The pigs received a complete vaccination programme. The farmer noticed that many of the nursery and grower pigs were constantly rubbing their heads and legs against the walls and doors of the pens. Some of these farm pens were starting to look highly polished. The itchy pig problem was mainly seen in the larger groups of nursery and grower-stage pigs. The farm workers stated that the affected pigs were bad tempered and irritable and that the scratching episodes were much worse whenever they smoked cigarettes near to the pigs. Closer examination of these affected pigs showed that they had waxy, dirty brown encrustations within their ears. The skin around their eyes and nose also seemed warm to touch, and was red and inflamed, with a dry crusty appearance and a noticeable bad smell (Fig. 11.1i). These affected pigs were also shaking their heads frequently, with some having enlarged blood-filled ears, known as aural haematomas. In some pigs with more long-standing and severe lesions, the crusty skin lesions extended down the neck and flanks (Fig. 11.1ii). The farm veterinarian collected numerous scrapings of the skin from the inner part of the ears. Portion of the scrapings were placed on to black paper for 5 min, the debris was blown off and a close examination showed several small light-coloured mites running around on the black paper.

Key Features

- Scratching and rubbing of head and ears.
- Crusty smelly lesions around and inside ears.

11.1a. What is this problem?
11.1b. What control measures may assist the herd?

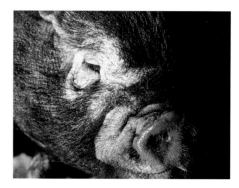

Fig. 11.1i. Crusty and itchy skin lesions on ears and face.

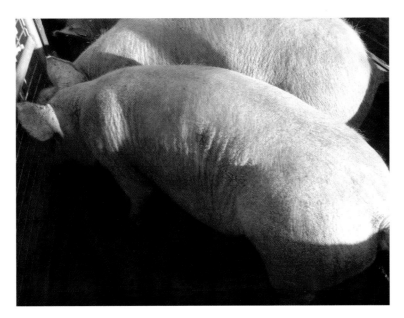

Fig. 11.1ii. Crusty and itchy skin lesions on ears and flanks of irritable pigs.

11.1 Comments

11.1a. The clinical signs and key features are typical of pig mange, due to the pig mange mite, *Sarcoptes scabei* var. *suis*. This disease is becoming less common, but it is still present on some farms. It is usually introduced to the farm when the farmer obtains an infected pig; incoming stock should carry a certificate and be checked to be clear of mange. The small *Sarcoptes* mange mite burrows into the skin of the pig and lays eggs within tunnels in the skin. This activity causes severe host irritation and the tremendous desire to scratch the skin. Portions of the ear scrapings can also be placed on to glass slides and mounted in 10% potassium hydroxide and examined at low power. Occasional microscopic parasites may be noted. The short legs and minute, round body of the mite detected in scrapings are typical of the pig mange mite, *S. scabei* var. *suis*. Conclusive diagnosis of swine scabies is not always easy to obtain because of the small size of the parasite and its location inside the skin. So the clinical picture and response to treatment must be closely examined.

11.1b. This mite continues to cause problems for the pig industry worldwide despite the availability of effective treatments, such as ivermectins. Eradication of mange from a pig farm can be reliably performed via two doses of ivermectin to all pigs on the farm and the use of pesticides to kill any mites in the environment. Pigs with mange may get ear haematomas, which are noticeable as a very swollen and distended ear lobe, with blood present under the skin of the affected ears. In general, open surgical repair of aural haematomas is not recommended, due to possible bacterial contamination during on-farm surgery. Healing of the lesion will occur over a few weeks to a 'cauliflower ear', reminiscent of those seen on rugby players.

11.2   Case Study

The farmer operated a small breeder and nursery pig farm, with some older-style wooden farm buildings, which had housed a range of breeding and growing pigs for many years (Fig. 11.2i). There were some other similar pig farms in the area and the farmer sometimes shared pig-farm equipment and building materials with these neighbourhood farms. The farmer noticed that several pigs, both adult pigs and young ones, within various pens appeared restless and were rubbing at their flanks. Some of the lactating sows appeared dull, depressed and slightly pale. Close examination of these affected pigs showed small but noticeable 6 mm long black insect parasites living on the areas of the pig with thin skin (i.e. on the flanks, shoulders, neck and the inner side of the legs) (Fig. 11.2ii). Some of these insects were in little groups. Very close examination of these adult insect parasites on the skin under a hand lens also showed some small pale egg-like structures nearby.

Key Features

- Pigs restless and dull and rubbing at their flanks on an older-style farm.
- Visible black insects on flanks of affected pigs.

11.2a. What is this problem?
11.2b. What control measures may assist the herd?

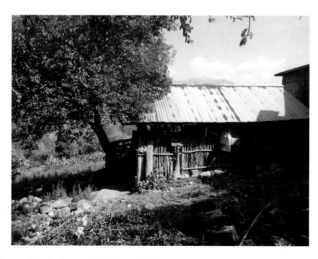

Fig. 11.2i. Older-style pig farm with shared farm equipment.

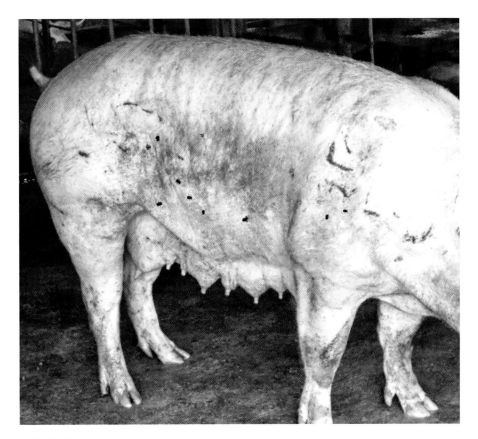

Fig. 11.2ii. Small black insects visible on flanks.

11.2 Comments

11.2a. These pigs are infected by *Haematopinus suis*, the giant pig louse. Lice are host-specific insects and so infections can only come from another pig. These lice do not transmit to humans or other animals. This disease is becoming less common, but it is still present on some smaller and older farms. It is usually introduced to the farm when the farmer buys or shares some farm materials or equipment, which are already infected with the lice or the small pale eggs, which are known as nits. The infected material may be items such as hay, troughs, old walls, fences, farm equipment or work clothes from other farms. The louse jumps on to the next pig and grips the hair on the skin with its claws, and moves along in a side-to-side fashion. Young lice (nymphs) spend much of their time in the ears of the pigs. As they mature, they move to the abdominal flank region. The *H. suis* louse burrows into skin veins and feeds exclusively on pig blood. Each louse lives on the pig for about 1 month and lays the nit eggs nearby.

11.2b. The pig louse is easily killed by modern products such as the ivermectins. Two injection treatments are given 10–14 days apart. It is important not to purchase materials from old pig farms that may be infected with lice or eggs.

11.3 Case Study

The farmer operated a large modern breeding farm, with normal farrowing rates and numbers of pigs born alive. The farmer was also expanding the herd with numerous gilts. The farrowing and lactation areas of the breeding farm were kept at a warm temperature to keep the pigs settled. The piglets in most litters were generally active and boisterous and appeared to be eating well. The farmer noticed an increasing problem in many litters of skin lesions in the older piglets. The affected piglets were generally between the ages of 10 and 40 days old. Close inspection of affected piglets and the recently weaned pigs showed a range of skin problems, which appeared to be the same problem at different stages of development. In some piglets, there were only a few dark brown and black small exudative scabby lesions on the face (Fig. 11.3i). In some other piglets, this had progressed to a stage where piglets had scabby, waxy, black lesions and dirty, greasy, crusty marks all around their eyes and head. The facial skin appeared to be more wrinkled with some thick dark greasy cracks. Most of these piglets did not appear to be particularly worried by their face lesions and tried to eat and run around normally. A few piglets with the worst lesions had these dark greasy lesions over most of their body (Fig. 11.3ii). These piglets were smelly and appeared to be dull and not eating properly. The farmer had injected a few piglets with antibiotics and ivermectin, but this did not help the piglets' condition.

Key Features

- Piglets affected at 10–40 days old.
- Dark brown-to-black, greasy, scabby lesions over the face.

11.3a. What is this problem?
11.3b. What control measures may assist the herd?

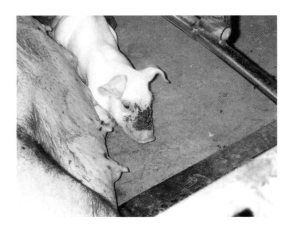

Fig. 11.3i. Piglet with mild greasy skin lesions.

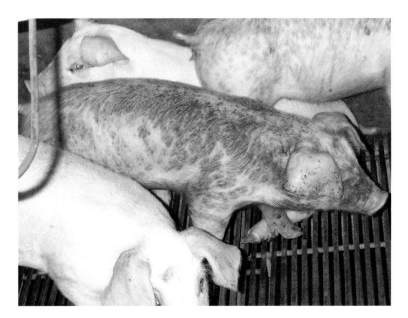

Fig. 11.3ii. Piglet with severe greasy skin lesions.

11.3 Comments

11.3a. The piglets in this breeding farm show typical signs of greasy pig disease. This is a bacterial infection of the skin caused by *Staphylococcus hyicus*. This is a common disease on all styles of pig farms around the world. There are no vaccines and the current treatments are not particularly effective. It affects pigs of all breeds. The disease is often worse in litters from gilts – presumably the piglets do not receive much protection against the infection from their mother's colostrum and milk. The disease is also worse in larger piglets that may be fighting among themselves and scratching their skin and allowing the bacterium to enter the skin. The disease will also occur more commonly where the farm does not perform teeth clipping in piglets. The entire sharp teeth damage the piglet skin and allow the bacterium to enter the skin. It will also occur more commonly if the farmer moves piglets around between litters, which will also increase fighting and damage to the piglet skin.

11.3b. For treatment of affected piglets, the piglet can be rinsed in a diluted disinfectant solution (e.g. chlorhexidine/cetrimide) and given penicillin injections. Most isolates of *S. hyicus* are penicillin-sensitive. On many farms, there is a poor response to these treatments and the disease seems to come and go over time. The problem can therefore be at a low level on many farms and specific control measures may not be justified on an economic basis. Some general control measures would include: (i) the checking of appropriate teeth-clipping procedures with clean and sharp equipment; and (ii) the removal of any straw or other sharp materials from the farrowing areas. It is also advised to wash and spray the piglets with a disinfectant solution at handling times such as processing at 4 days old and at weaning time. If the problem is serious, then piglets can also be injected with a long-acting antibiotic at 4 days old.

11.4 Case Study

The farmer operated a large modern breeding farm in an isolated location. The farm was expanding and a large number of new gilts had recently been purchased from a major commercial supplier of modern genetic lines of female pigs. These new gilts had excellent health certificates and were mixed in the same breeding areas as the previous farm sows. The farm was free of parasites such as worms, mites and lice. The farm had no serious problems with diarrhoea or coughing pigs. The farmer noticed that his new gilts developed some problems around farrowing and lactation periods. The gilts appeared thin and pale (Fig. 11.4i) and had a low colostrum and milk yield, with reduced numbers of pigs weaned. Close inspection indicated that the gilts were dull and inactive and their skin was pale across their body. This was confirmed by examination of the areas inside their eyelids (known as the sclera), which were pale and white. The farm veterinarian took some blood from these pigs and made thin smears of the blood on some glass slides. These blood films were fixed in methanol and stained by routine blood stains, such as the Giemsa stain (Fig. 11.4ii). Careful examination of these blood smears showed many red cells had detectable small bacteria agents that were 1 μm in diameter, compared with the overall cell size of 7 μm diameter. The farm veterinarian also performed standard blood tests, such as red cell counts.

Key Features

- Groups of pale depressed pigs.
- Blood smears show distinctive bacteria on the red blood cells.

11.4a. What is this problem?
11.4b. What control measures may assist the herd?

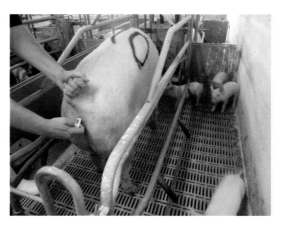

Fig. 11.4i. Pale depressed gilts in farrowing areas.

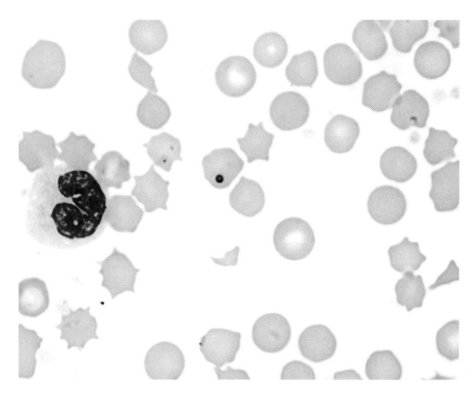

Fig. 11.4ii. Photograph of blood smear from an affected pig.

11.4 Comments

11.4a. This is anaemia caused by the small bacterium, *Mycoplasma suis*. The bacteria infect the red blood cells, disrupting them so they break up easily. This leads to a lack of proper red blood cells and reduced oxygen moving around the body of the pigs. The anaemia can be confirmed by checking the blood values of the affected pigs compared with the values in normal pigs. Typically in *M. suis* infections, the red cell counts are very low, such as $4.2–5.5 \times 10^6$ cells/mm^3 of blood, compared with a suggested normal range of $5.6–9.5 \times 10^6$ cells/mm^3. This disease occurs on sporadic occasions in all types of pig farming systems, including modern farms. It occurs more commonly in large groups of pigs kept in close contact, where blood from infected pigs may be shared with other pigs. This can occur where farms use the same needles and syringes and farm equipment among different pigs. This may act to spread the disease from one infected group of pigs to another, such as the new and old breeding pigs on the farm in this case study.

11.4b. The bacteria and the disease are easily treated by injection of the pigs with a suitable antibiotic, such as oxytetracycline. There are no vaccines. The disease can also be limited by use of good hygiene of equipment and making sure that fresh needles are used for all pigs, at injection times such as late pregnancy vaccination schedules. Over time, groups of pigs typically develop immunity to the bacteria and the actual disease condition fades.

11.5   Case Study

The farmer operated an established medium-sized breeder, nursery and finisher farm system. There had been many different sources of pigs to the farm over the years, with various age groups and breeds now present on the farm. The farmer had experienced a range of disease problems, with high mortality among weaner pigs, many coughing pigs and other ongoing health issues. The farmer therefore used a lot of pig treatments, but he was concerned about farm costs and did not use many commercial vaccines. The farmer noticed that several grower and finisher pigs scattered around the farm had skin lesions. Close inspection indicated highly noticeable, dark red-to-dark purple, roughly circular lesions about 1 cm in diameter present over the hindquarters of these affected pigs (Fig. 11.5i). The lesions were visible on the perineum area, the top of the hind legs, extending in some pigs further forward on the trunk. The pigs were dull and appeared to be losing weight slowly. The lymph nodes of the pigs appear to be enlarged (Fig. 11.5ii), and the inguinal lymph nodes could be easily palpated and visible.

Key Features

- Older grower and finisher pigs affected.
- Dark red–purple circular lesions over the hindquarters.

11.5a. What is this problem?
11.5b. What control measures may assist the herd?

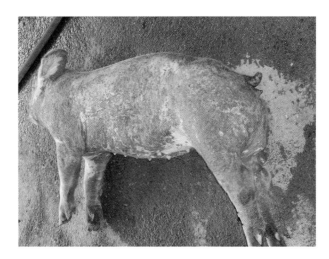

Fig. 11.5i. Purple skin patches over the hindquarter regions of a pig.

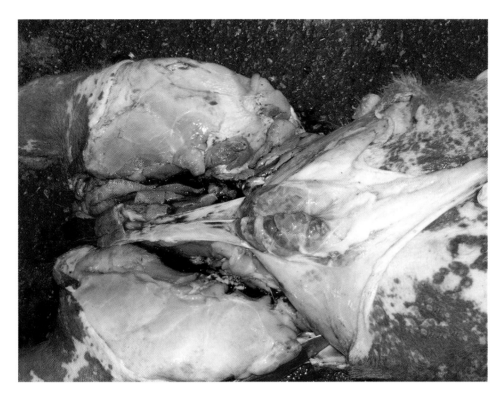

Fig. 11.5ii. Autopsy of a case of skin lesions with enlarged lymph nodes.

11.5 Comments

11.5a. These pigs show typical signs of the porcine dermatopathy and nephropathy syndrome, known as PDNS. This syndrome is closely associated with the presence of active PCV-2 infection. It is thought to be an aberrant immune response to infection by this virus, within the pig. The affected pigs may also have considerable damage to their kidneys. The lymph node enlargement around the body of the pig is a typical sign of active PCV-2 infection. PDNS is not particularly common, even in herds with active PCV-2 infections, but it is a highly visible disease syndrome and affected pigs are easily noticed. Cases are usually sporadic with only a few pigs affected around the farm at any time.

11.5b. The pigs do not respond to treatment and should be culled. PCV-2 infection and its associated disease issues, such as PDNS, have been dramatically brought under control in pig populations in the past 10 years, by the introduction of effective commercial vaccines. The incidence of PDNS has therefore reduced greatly. The cases presented on this farm are therefore due to the farmer failing to use PCV-2 vaccines in a proper manner. All farmers are urged to add PCV-2 vaccines to their vaccine list, as they are highly beneficial to the profitability of pig farming, when applied to the pigs appropriately.

11.6 Case Study

The farmer operated a large farm system with breeding farms linked to production pig grow-out (nursery and finisher) facilities. The breeding pigs and young piglets were fully vaccinated with commercial vaccines. The weaned pigs moved to separate weaner-to-finisher production pig sites at 3–4 weeks old. The farm system did have problems with sickness and diarrhoea in the weaner nursery areas on these grow-out sites in batches of weaned pigs arriving from the breeding farms. The problems began soon after weaning at 3–4 weeks old. Some of these pigs had died and the overall mortality rate in the weaner groups was high. Close inspection showed many sick and dehydrated weaner pigs in the affected pens, and some weaner pigs with yellow diarrhoea. The ears and snouts of many of these sick pigs had moderate dark red-to-purple discoloration (known as cyanosis) (Fig. 11.6i). The skin of some of the pigs also had some dark blotchy patches over the stomach and legs. The tips of the ears of some pigs appeared very dark and shrunken. At autopsy of some of these pigs, the farmer and veterinarian noticed that there was also dark red-to-purple discoloration over the stomach of the pig and the small intestines were dilated and reddened with fluid intestinal contents (Fig. 11.6ii).

Key Features

- Dark purple skin colour (cyanosis) over the ears, snout and legs.
- Weaner pig illness and deaths.

11.6a. What is this problem?
11.6b. What control measures may assist the herd?

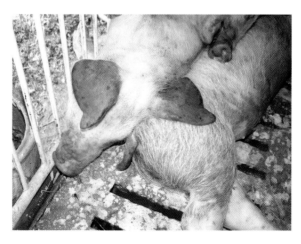

Fig. 11.6i. Sick weaner pigs with dark ears and snouts.

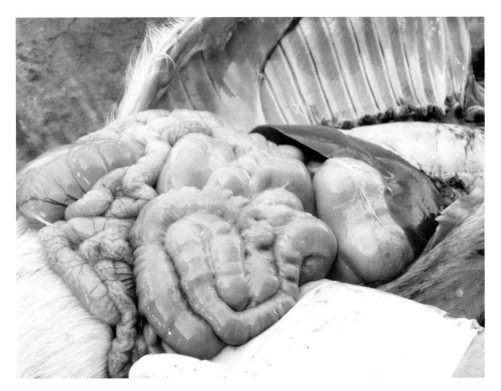

Fig. 11.6ii. Autopsy of pig with dark ears and snout indicates gastrointestinal lesions.

11.6 Comments

11.6a. The skin findings in these pigs are a mild to moderate form of cyanosis. The purple and dark red blotchy areas are due to congestion of blood in areas of the skin and stomach. These changes are only a secondary event and are always associated with a more serious primary event, such as a typical blood poisoning case (septicaemia), a swine fever or an enteric disease such as colibacillosis. It is therefore important to look beyond this common finding of red and purple discoloration of the skin and look deeper into the history and autopsy and other findings to discover the true cause of the problems in the pigs. In pigs with colibacillosis, an enterotoxigenic *Escherichia coli* (ETEC) colonizes the pigs' intestines shortly after weaning, causing yellow diarrhoea and these skin changes. Results from a bacteriology laboratory can confirm a bacterial culture of *E. coli* from fresh intestine samples.

11.6b. *E. coli* and the ETEC strains are a common background organism that is considered to be 'embedded' in most pig farms, presumably in faecal materials in the pens, walkways and slurry. This embedded nature explains its constant occurrence and outbreaks when appropriate control measures are not taken. The occurrence of clinical ETEC infections in post-weaned pigs had dropped away to a very low level since the 1980s with the introduction of in-feed zinc oxide at sufficient pharmaceutical levels (1500–3000 ppm) in early starter diets. However, some government initiatives aimed at environmental cleanliness have now led to limits in its general use, and hence an increase in intestine cases like this study, with the prominent skin and stomach congestion.

11.7   Case Study

The farmer operated a large farm system with several breeder farms and nursery and finisher sites. The farmer and his technical team planned the various vaccine and medication programmes. The local staff at each farm site performed the actual handling of the breeder and finisher pigs, at the specified times when they were given their vaccines and medications. The farmer preferred to use injection methods to give vaccines and medications to large groups of pigs (Fig. 11.7i). So the staff had been given instructions on how to handle and inject pigs with the full and proper amount of commercial product into the muscle tissues. They had also been instructed to inject away from the valuable parts of the pig such as the back and leg muscles. On one farm unit, many pigs were observed to have noticeable lumps in the skin of their neck (Fig. 11.7ii). In the other units, lumps were evident on only the occasional pig. Close inspection of the necks of the affected pigs showed that the lumps were 2–5 cm in diameter and raised above the skin surface. The lumps were very firm and painful to the pig when they were touched. In some pigs, the skin over the centre of the lumps had become ulcerated, with the formation of a dark scab.

Key Features

- Older grower pigs and adults affected.
- Firm, raised, ulcerated lesions in the centre of the neck.

11.7a. What is this problem?
11.7b. What control measures may assist the herd?

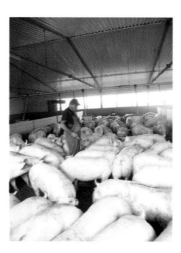

Fig. 11.7i. Injection programme for many pigs.

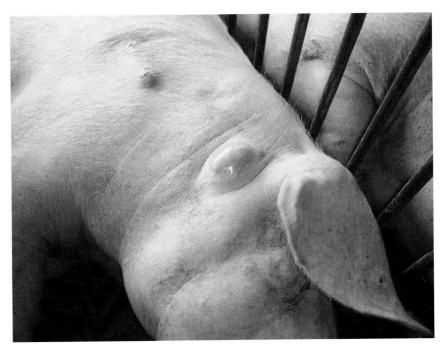

Fig. 11.7ii. Pig with noticable injection-site lumps in the neck.

11.7 Comments

11.7a. These pigs show typical signs of injection-site reactions and infections. Pig farms and pig pens are dirty contaminated environments. When a single syringe and needle is used on many pigs in a pen, there is the strong possibility to collect environmental bacteria on the needle. When that needle is used again on the next pig, then these environmental bacteria can be injected directly into the pig tissue. These bacteria can then set up a local inflammation reaction and create a lump. This type of needle contamination is more likely when injecting pigs that are in groups and when pigs are bigger and more active. This situation means that the farm worker is under more pressure and needles are more likely to become contaminated on pen walls and floors.

11.7b. Injections of groups of pigs is a difficult and dangerous job. It is important to perform this job with well-trained people working in a team, who can assist each other at all times. Farm workers can be pushed over, or accidentally inject themselves, or become injured in farm pens and gates in these situations. If a pig moves during the injection, there is also a major risk of the possible situation to leave some part of a broken needle inside the pig muscle. Any pig that has part of a broken needle retained in its muscle must be clearly identified for the rest of its life, so a consumer of pork can never eat the needle.

Injection programmes in groups of pigs can also lead to the unwanted transmission of blood-borne diseases, such as PRRS. Blood may be taken up in the injection needle of one pig and carried directly to the next pig that is injected. It is therefore important to change needles frequently when pigs are given injections.

Skin and Muscle Problems in Pigs

11.8   Case Study

The farmer operated a large established breeder farm, with various older buildings. The sows and gilts were kept in groups in pens, when they were not pregnant. After the female pigs were mated, they were moved into individual stalls for the early gestation, farrowing and lactation periods. These pigs in stalls were kept cool in the hot summer months, with lines of dripping water on to their backs. The farmer had expanded the sow herd with the purchase of many new lines of well-muscled lean meat breeds over the past years. He had also replaced some of the older-style farrowing and lactation stalls on concrete floors with new moulded-plastic floors. The farmer noticed that many of the sows and gilts in the later stages of the farrowing and lactation period had developed open rough skin wounds and sores over the area of their shoulders (Fig. 11.8i). The sores appeared on pigs housed both in stalls located on concrete floors and in pigs housed in stalls on the new plastic floors. The sores had become more open and ulcerated in pigs that appeared in thin body condition. The farmer had applied some sprays to the wounds, but they did not heal spontaneously and persisted for several weeks (Fig. 11.8ii).

Key Features

- Thin sows in the farrowing area.
- Large persistent sores on the shoulder area.

11.8a. What is this problem?
11.8b. What control measures may assist the herd?

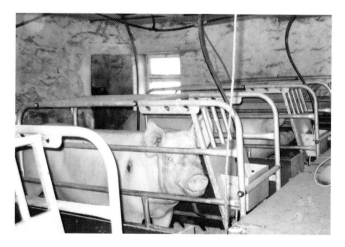

Fig. 11.8i. Thin sows in farrowing areas with shoulder sores.

11.8 Comments

11.8a. These skin ulcers are known as shoulder sores. The sores develop when the pig rubs its shoulder blade bone against the floor when it is lying down and when it is trying to get up. They commonly appear in female pigs around 3 weeks after the farrowing date, towards the end of the lactation period. The most severe lesions occur at this time because this is when pigs have lost condition and are thinnest, with the shoulder blade bone at its most prominent. Shoulder sores have become more common due to the popular choices of breed lines of pigs with greater growth rates and lean meat. The females of these lean breeds tend to have little subcutaneous fat and so the shoulder bone is more prominent. As the sow goes through lactation, the limited fat in this area is burned up, so the underlying shoulder bone becomes more prominent and prone to damage. After periods of damage to this area, blood flow to the sore stops and the skin dies and ulcerates. This problem occurs in sows kept on old, rough concrete and metal floors, which will abrade the skin. It is also seen commonly on modern moulded-plastic floors. This is probably because the slippery nature of these floors means that the sow must push about trying to stand up and so cause the damage to the shoulder skin area.

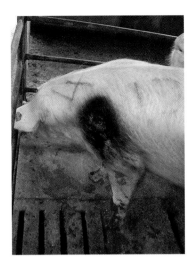

Fig. 11.8ii. Thin sow with ulcerated and persistent shoulder sore.

11.8b. The treatment of affected pigs in lactation may involve antibiotics and anti-inflammatory medicines. Usually the situation of an affected sow can also be improved by adding carpet or mat or other soft materials to the stalls and directly to the sow. Where rough concrete or metals are present on floors, they can be repaired and improved by applications of a smooth rubber coating. If sows are having difficulty on slippery plastic floors, then safety mats can be added to the floors. However, the use of mats in stall areas means that removal of faeces and urine is more difficult and the area can become dirty.

The prevention of new cases requires that sow nutrition is kept at optimum levels from the earliest stages as a gilt, to maintain the most possible subcutaneous fat. The sow must then be fed as much as possible in the farrowing house, with attention to methods of feeding and amounts offered.

11.9   Case Study

The farmer operated a finisher pig farm and an adjacent slaughterhouse facility. The slaughterhouse also received pigs from other local farms. Groups of pigs were unloaded from trucks and often kept in some holding sheds prior to entering the slaughter facility. These holding sheds were fully enclosed with numerous pens where pigs were kept without exercise or movements. The pens were constantly damp due to a mixture of pig urine, water showers, cleaning sprays, disinfectant usage and a concrete floor environment. Some pens had better drainage than others. The slaughterhouse facility was busy, so some groups of finisher pigs were housed overnight in these damp holding sheds (Fig. 11.9i). The farmer noticed that when pigs were held in these pens in these holding sheds for long periods, they developed bright red patches of skin over the back of their hind legs. These skin lesions were also visible when the pigs were taken inside the slaughter facility. The skin lesions seemed to be worse in pigs from some farm trucks and when pigs are kept sitting and sleeping for long periods (more than 4 h) in the damp pens in the holding sheds. Close inspection showed that the skin lesions were a red rash on the skin of the back surface of the hind leg hams of all pigs (Fig. 11.9ii). The skin lesions were superficial and did not affect deeper meat quality.

Key Features

- Pigs sitting in wet urine and disinfectant for long periods.
- Bright red scald skin on the back of the legs.

11.9a. What is this problem?
11.9b. What control measures may assist the herd?

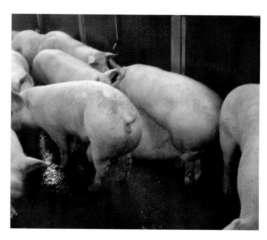

Fig. 11.9i. Groups of pigs sitting in wet, urine-soaked environment.

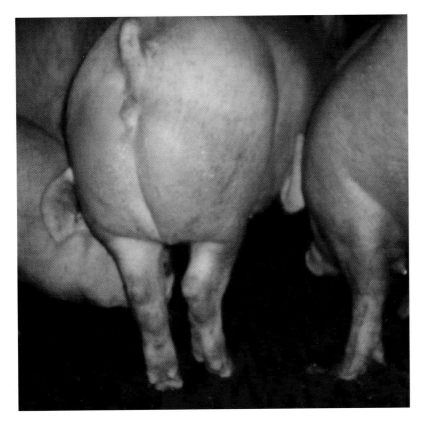

Fig. 11.9ii. Superficial red skin rash on the back of the legs.

11.9 Comments

11.9a. This is scalding of the skin, which occurs when pigs sit for long periods on wet and damp floors soaked with urine, sometimes known as urine scald. It may be exacerbated if there is also some irritant disinfectant present in the urine-and-water mixture on the floors. This soaking environment and any minor skin abrasion damages the skin surface to form the visible red, congested rash. The situations where pigs are forced to sit in wet urine-soaked floors can include holding pens, as in this case. Urine scald can also occur when sows are housed in stalls and pens with solid concrete floors, where the drainage is poor and urine accumulates on the floor where the sow is resting. This reaction of soaking pig urine and skin is known to provoke a strong irritant reaction in the skin in some situations. The bright red skin scald noted on the rear and hind legs of pigs or sows that have spent periods sitting in urine-soaked floors is distinctive.

11.9b. It is important to allow pigs in confined spaces the ability to move around to dry well-drained areas that do not contain urine or disinfectant on the floor areas. Many disinfectants are strong chemicals that can irritate the skin of pigs. It is therefore important that when disinfectant is used it is washed away and the area on the truck or pens is rinsed properly.

11.10   Case Study

A large rural village had numerous pigs moving around between the houses and shops. The pigs were scavengers and consumed waste products from homes and restaurants (Fig. 11.10i). The village also had many local rats and mice. Some of the village families slaughtered some of the older village pigs at festival times and prepared various sausages and dry meat dishes. Some members of these families developed clinical signs of muscle weakness, swelling of the face and high fevers. The village pigs appeared relatively normal, but as part of the investigation, the next pigs to be slaughtered were examined and inspected for parasites.

Close inspection indicated that there were white streaks in some muscle fibres from the tongue, rib and diaphragm muscles. Portions of these muscles were taken from the pigs and placed directly under a microscope. In some areas of these white-streaked muscles, larval forms inside small cysts were noted (Fig. 11.10ii).

Key Features

- Normal pigs in village and backyard settings.
- Illness in humans consuming raw pork.
- Microscopic parasites in pork muscle.

11.10a. What is this problem?
11.10b. What control procedures can be used?

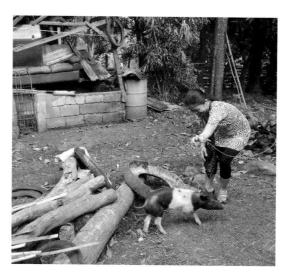

Fig. 11.10i. Village pigs eating waste food products.

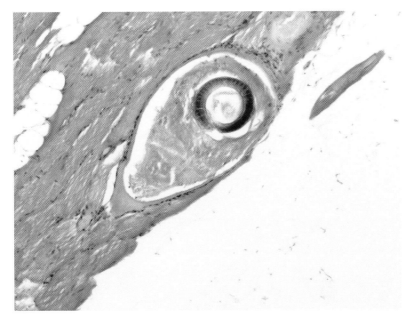

Fig. 11.10ii. Worm larva inside a cyst in pig muscle.

11.10　Comments

11.10a. This is *Trichinella spiralis*, the muscle nematode, which infects pigs, rodents and carnivorous mammals, including humans. After ingesting infected muscle, the digestive enzymes of the stomach liberate the larvae from their cysts. These larvae then develop in the intestine to become adult worms, only 3–4 mm long. These adult worms produce active larvae which pass to the pork muscles via the bloodstream. In the muscles the larvae grow and curl up into a spiral coil within a cyst. These muscle cysts can persist for a long time or they may die and become mineralized.

　T. spiralis has little effect on infected pigs, apart from the white streaks in some muscles, but it is important from a public-health point of view. It is one reason why pork is not favoured in some societies. The most characteristic symptoms of human trichinosis are high fever, muscle weakness and swelling (oedema) of the face and eyelids. Nervous signs include confusion, dizziness and paresis. Pigs and humans with trichinella usually have raised counts of eosinophil blood cells and raised levels of the muscle enzyme, creatine kinase.

11.10b. Many countries have regulations to examine the pork muscles from slaughter pigs for this parasite, to ensure it does not enter the food chain. It is important to cook pork fully, because smoking, salting and drying are not effective at killing these tough nematode cysts.

　The control of rats in villages and pig farms is important, as these rodents can transmit the parasite in their muscles – they will both eat dead pigs left in the open and also they will be eaten themselves by pigs. It is also important not to leave dead pigs in a place where they can be eaten by other pigs – pigs will readily become cannibals and may consume infected muscle from other pigs.

11.11   Case Study

A rural village had groups of open-range pigs of various ages running around between the houses (Fig. 11.11i). The village and the surrounding rural areas did not have an official public toilet or human sewage waste system. Many houses in the village did not have any covered tank or other device for completely retaining the human sewage waste. The pigs were kept around the village for scavenging food scraps and other waste materials. A few of the village pigs appeared to be dull, with some muscle stiffness and reluctance to move. On some occasions, a few of the larger village pigs were herded to a local butcher for slaughter and production of pork for consumption. At the slaughter process, numerous small cysts were noted in the pig meat. Close inspection indicated several white-to-yellow, pearl-shaped, firm, tough nodules scattered in the pig muscle tissues (Fig. 11.11ii). These pearl-shaped nodules were particularly apparent in the tongue and shoulder pork muscle areas.

Key Features

- Village pigs with access to human sewage.
- Pearl-shaped parasite nodules in pork.

11.11a. What is this problem?
11.11b. What control procedures can be used?

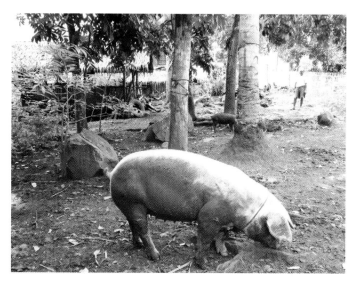

Fig. 11.11i. Rural village pigs.

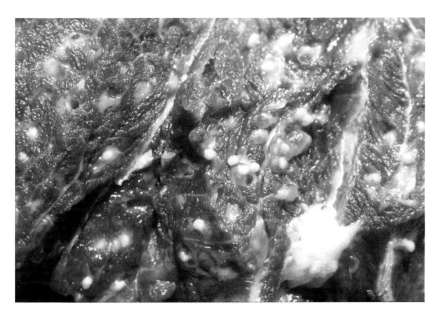

Fig. 11.11ii. Pearl-shaped nodules in pork muscle.

11.11 Comments

11.11a. This is pearly pork – it is due to a parasite called *Cysticercus cellulosae* found in pig muscle. This is the intermediate stage of the tapeworm *Taenia solium*. This tapeworm occurs in the small intestine of humans, so it is a two-host parasite, pigs and humans. After ingestion of infected pork by humans, the larvae emerge and attach to the initial part of the intestine for development. The tapeworm can become a 2–4 m long adult stage of *T. solium* in the human intestine. The most frequent form of transmission of the tapeworm to pigs is when tapeworm eggs are present in human faeces, which is not properly disposed of. The infected human faeces are then eaten by the scavenging pigs. The larvae hatch when the eggs appear inside the pig intestine and they further migrate to the pork muscle, but also to other organs. These muscle cysts develop over 2–3 months. These cysts have a tough fibrotic wall and contain a small tapeworm head, known as a scolex. In pigs infected by pearly pork parasites, fever and muscle stiffness may be noted.

The adult *Taenia* tapeworm in humans causes few clinical signs. However, infection of the brain arising from self-infection with eggs and the larval form of cysticercus within humans is manifested with headache, dizziness, hydrocephalus, loss of vision and nausea. These damaging nervous signs are a common and often fatal outcome in affected regions.

11.11b. This disease remains common in pig-raising areas of the world, where pigs and humans are kept in close proximity in rural settings. Consumers of pork must be aware and avoid any muscle parasite cysts. The main factor for control of this disease is the prevention of access of pigs to human faeces, therefore this must be strongly avoided. Human faeces sewage systems should be closed to village or household pigs. Farm workers must be reminded never to defecate inside open pig-holding areas and therefore must be provided with a working toilet.

11.12   Case Study

The farmer operated an established medium-sized breeder, nursery and finisher farm system with buildings and some open-pasture pens. He had further developed these outdoor spaces for pigs and usually moved groups of breeding and growing pigs from the buildings to these outdoor pens, in the early summer (Fig. 11.12i). The farmer provided plenty of feed and water outlets for the outdoor pigs, but there was no shade or trees and the pasture ground was firm. The weather went through a long hot and sunny spell in the period after the pigs went to these outdoor spaces. The farmer noticed that many pigs developed a reddening of the skin over the ears and back. Over some weeks, he noticed that some pigs developed more severe problems with areas of red rashes and some blisters in these exposed skin areas. Close inspection indicated that some of these pigs appeared to be in pain – they squealed a lot and dipped their back down. Some pigs were seen occasionally to drop on to their stomach and then get up, when they were moving around the pastures. Close inspection also indicated that areas of skin over the ears and back were bright red and hot and painful to touch (Fig. 11.12ii). Some areas of skin on the back were rough and peeling. The appetite of the pigs was poor and they were in poor body condition. Some of the pregnant pigs in the outdoor breeder pig groups had spontaneous abortions of their litters.

Key Features

- Pigs placed into sunny outdoor farm areas.
- Red rash over the back and ears.

11.12a. What is this problem?
11.12b. What control procedures can be used?

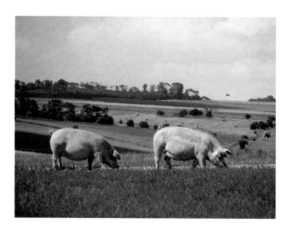

Fig. 11.12i. Open-range pigs in sunny pastures.

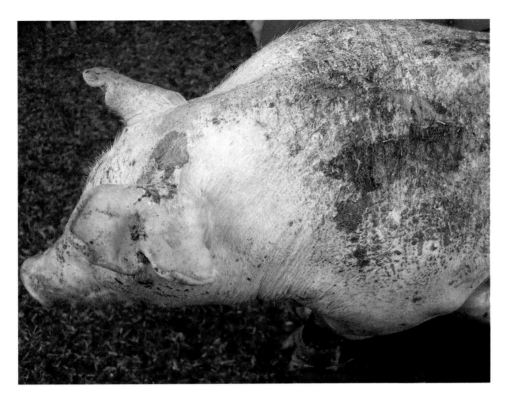

Fig. 11.12ii. Rough reddened skin on the back and ears.

11.12 Comments

11.12a. This is sunburn of the exposed skin in pigs. It is analogous to sunburn in humans, with exposed pink skin being the most susceptible. It is seen most commonly when pigs such as gilts or finishers are placed into open sunshine areas in early summer, in northern summer months such as May or June. As well as the obvious skin problems, it can lead to depression of appetite, abortions and reduced farrowing rates.

11.12b. Pigs that are severely sunburnt should be placed in the shade and an emollient suntan cream can be applied to the back. The pigs should also be given injections of painkillers. Where pigs are facing sunburn problems, then they may be cooled with a water spray or a pool, but this will not protect them against further sunburn. To prevent and control sunburn, pigs should be provided with shade areas, such as open-sided sheds. However, this is not useful for lactating sows with litters, as the sows will lie in the shade and neglect the piglets. The use of outdoor areas for raising pigs needs to consider the various health and management problems specific to this form of pig farming. Besides sunburn, outdoor pigs and piglets will also be much more likely to suffer thefts and attack by predator carnivores, such as foxes.

Index